A WOMAN'S
Guide to DIABETES
A PATH TO WELLNESS

BRANDY BARNES, MSW, & NATALIE STRAND, MD

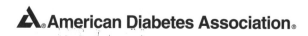
American Diabetes Association.

Director, Book Publishing, Abe Ogden; *Managing Editor*, Greg Guthrie; *Acquisitions Editor*, Victor Van Beuren; *Project Manager*, Wendy Martin-Shuma; *Production Manager*, Melissa Sprott; *Composition*, Naylor Design, Inc.; *Cover Design*, Vis-à-Vis Creative, Inc.; *Cover Photographer*, Kelly Campbell; *Printer*, Versa Press.

Printed in the United States of America
1 3 5 7 9 10 8 6 4 2

The suggestions and information contained in this publication are generally consistent with the *Clinical Practice Recommendations* and other policies of the American Diabetes Association, but they do not represent the policy or position of the Association or any of its boards or committees. Reasonable steps have been taken to ensure the accuracy of the information presented. However, the American Diabetes Association cannot ensure the safety or efficacy of any product or service described in this publication. Individuals are advised to consult a physician or other appropriate health care professional before undertaking any diet or exercise program or taking any medication referred to in this publication. Professionals must use and apply their own professional judgment, experience, and training and should not rely solely on the information contained in this publication before prescribing any diet, exercise, or medication. The American Diabetes Association—its officers, directors, employees, volunteers, and members—assumes no responsibility or liability for personal or other injury, loss, or damage that may result from the suggestions or information in this publication.

♾ The paper in this publication meets the requirements of the ANSI Standard Z39.48-1992 (permanence of paper).

ADA titles may be purchased for business or promotional use or for special sales. To purchase more than 50 copies of this book at a discount, or for custom editions of this book with your logo, contact the American Diabetes Association at the address below or at booksales@diabetes.org.

American Diabetes Association
1701 North Beauregard Street
Alexandria, Virginia 22311
DOI: 10.2337/9781580405294

Library of Congress Cataloging-in-Publication Data

Strand, Natalie.
  A woman's guide to diabetes : a path to wellness / Natalie Strand and Brandy Barnes.
  pages cm
  Includes bibliographical references and index.
  ISBN 978-1-58040-529-4 (alk. paper)
  1. Diabetes in women. 2. Mind and body. 3. Women—Health and hygiene. I. Barnes, Brandy. II. Title.
  RC660.4.S77 2014
  616.4'620082--dc23
  2014001430

TABLE OF CONTENTS

PREFACE

As women with diabetes, we strongly believe that life should be celebrated, not *in spite of* diabetes, but *in light of* diabetes. From the days we each were diagnosed, we have made it our missions to not allow diabetes to stop us from doing anything. We hope to help you adopt the same outlook, if you haven't already. Consider this: If you are a woman with diabetes, you have already amassed an incredible amount of experience that your peers without diabetes simply do not have. We're not just talking about your diabetes knowledge, but also your multi-tasking, stress-management and endurance-building experience. In a sense, diabetes gives you an advantage in life . . . if you view it from the right perspective.

When we came together to write this book, we had only known each other a few months, but our diabetes diagnoses bonded us immediately. We talked about a myriad of diabetes-related topics that made us feel heard and understood: We *had* to be long-lost sisters! *Diabetes* sisters, that is! We shared a passion for empowering women, a desire to help women better understand how to flourish with diabetes, and a concern for the lack of information (and for the misinformation) that was available to women with diabetes. In addition, both of us were diagnosed with diabetes in our teen years and we now are in our 30s.

We have our share of differences as well. While one of us lives in the hustle and bustle of Los Angeles, California, practicing medicine, the other lives in a quiet suburb of Durham, North Carolina, running a national nonprofit organization. We have very different personalities: One of us is more free-spirited and the other, more serious. A big part of *"owning"* your diabetes is opening up and being willing to share with and learn from others, including those who can provide you with different perspectives, as we have. We encourage you to open your mind to the different experiences and perspectives provided in this book.

To say that we are proud of this book would be an understatement. It was written from a place of passion, determination, understanding, and concern. We intend not only to make you feel good about yourself and learn a lot, but also to broach some difficult or challenging issues that may make you uncomfortable. (Just know that discomfort is a sign of growth!) You're going to read about topics ranging from "diabetes guilt" to traveling with diabetes. You may read about some things that sound scary or depressing, but you will also laugh at our diabetes mishaps and uncover some new information to help you better manage your diabetes.

There will be points throughout the book where you will be asked to write down your thoughts: Turning inward may be the hardest part of your transformation, but it is vitally important that you understand yourself as you make this journey. We want you to identify and enhance the strengths you already have as a result of your diabetes. At the conclusion of the book, we hope you are more knowledgeable and informed about female-specific diabetes issues, uplifted through our personal stories, and transformed in the way you view yourself as a woman with diabetes.

Most of all, we hope you learn that you are not alone with this disease. There are millions of other women with diabetes just like you who are going through the same challenges.

If up until this point you have just been surviving with diabetes, it's time for a change. It's time to start *thriving* with diabetes. We want this to be a book that enables you to do whatever it takes to live a happy, healthy, and proud life as a strong woman with diabetes. Let's get started!

Natalie Strand, MD   *Brandy Barnes, MSW*

GUIDE TO THE JOURNALING SECTIONS

 NOTES ON MY JOURNEY: Record valuable information that you're learning from the book

 SOUL-SEARCHING: Answer questions and complete various activities designed to help you reflect more deeply on your feelings and/or struggles

LIFE APPLICATION: Record specific steps you will take to address your personal health

 MY DIABETES JOURNAL: Use these "guided journaling" sections to gain valuable insight about your behavior and emotions

ACKNOWLEDGMENTS

NATALIE SAYS...

I would like to take this opportunity to thank the many people in my life who have helped me live passionately, fully, and at peace with my diabetes. I would like to thank my family, for your strength during my diagnosis and for your support as I sometimes trip over the hurdles that life presents to me. To my dad, thank you for being an example of how to follow your dreams, no matter how big they are. To my brother, you have inspired me by your strength and character during your own diagnosis with diabetes. To my mom, thank you for pushing me to be my best. To Carolyn, you changed my life. You said "yes" when others said "no." To Dr. Anne Peters, you have set the standard of how a physician should treat patients. Thank you for helping me in every facet of my diabetes and life. To my husband, thank you for caring an unbelievable amount about my overall health and wellness. Thank you for measuring out the carbs in the breakfasts that you often make for me. You motivate me to take the best care of myself possible.

To my friends, who are also my family, thank you for always listening to me. Thank you for not letting diabetes scare you away from sharing in crazy adventures with me. From *The Amazing Race* to cross-country road trips, you have been by my side for incredible highs and lows (pun intended). To the diabetes community, which is also an extension of my family, thank you for welcoming me with open arms. Thank you for all the "beeping" you do when we are in a room together; you make me feel at home. Thank you for the support, education, and friendship.

To Brandy, thank you for all you do. Thank you for helping me turn my dream of writing a book for women with diabetes into a reality. And to diabetes, thank you for making me the woman I am. Without you, many of my favorite parts of life would not exist.

BRANDY SAYS...

As with any major project, it takes a great team to make all the elements come together in a book. I want to extend my personal and sincere thanks to many people, for without them this book would not exist. First and foremost, I thank God for giving meaning to my life through diabetes. I also want to thank John Buse, MD, PhD, for always encouraging me to be a "diabetes pioneer" and for showing me repeatedly that diabetes should not dim the dreams I have for my life. I cannot give enough praise and thanks for Anna Norton and all of my new friends and "sisters" I have met through DiabetesSisters because they have provided the backdrop for so much of this book. I also want to thank the numerous lifelong friends I have met through the Diabetes Online Community (DOC). You kept me grounded!

I thank my entire family for never viewing me as a "diabetic" but rather as "Brandy, who happens to have diabetes." I see now how instrumental their view was in shaping my view of myself and what I could accomplish in life. To my parents, Dennis and Debbie Carver, I thank you for teaching me to persevere through life's many obstacles. This set the stage early on for me to view diabetes as simply another one of life's obstacles to overcome. To my sister, Candace, I thank you for showing me what true sisterhood is all about and for taking the time to really understand what my life is like as a woman with diabetes.

To Natalie, I will be forever grateful for your friendship and willingness to tackle such a big project like this with me. You represent true "diabetes sisterhood"!

Most importantly, I thank my husband, Chris, and my daughter, Summer, for their steadfast support and unconditional love. Chris, thank you for encouraging me to follow God's plan and pursue my passion. You are my rock! Summer, you are my inspiration and the main reason I want to make the world a better place. Thank you for reminding me to stop, smell the roses, and be grateful for the simple beauty that exists in everyday life. Your unwavering enthusiasm and constant encouragement mean more than you will ever know.

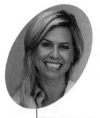

Back to Basics

NATALIE SAYS...

For many 12-year-old girls, the summer before middle school is a really important time. It's when they start to feel like grown-ups. I spent that summer wondering about more than what my new school would be like, because that was the summer I was diagnosed with diabetes.

I had all of the classic symptoms, but at the time, no one was looking for them. I had to use the restroom all the time. I was always thirsty. Even though I was skin and bones, I was rapidly losing weight. My legs were cramping severely from dehydration.

One weekend I escaped the Arizona heat by heading to a camp in the woods with a local group. I became pretty well known among the other campers. Because I was so thirsty, I was drinking soda at such an impressive rate that I built an enormous pyramid with the empty cans in my bunk. By the time I returned home just 2 days later, I was definitely feeling and looking a lot worse.

When my parents picked me up, they took one look at me and knew that something was very wrong. My dad is a physician, and he was suspicious enough to buy keto sticks from the local pharmacy to test my urine for ketones. I tested positive, and he instantly knew that I had diabetes. He told me that I had to pack up and get ready for a trip to the hospital. Back then (in 1990), a diabetes diagnosis required an almost 2-week hospital stay! As I was getting ready to go to the hospital, I remember gazing over at a large bag of gummy bears that I had stashed in my bedroom. My 12-year-old mind worried that I would never be able to have those gummy bears again. Looking back as an adult, I have to laugh at the fact that this was my biggest concern!

The following weeks changed my life. I went from being a carefree preteen to learning about meal exchanges, insulin shots, and blood sugar testing. It was such a whirlwind of information. Some of it was exciting (I get to carry a purse to school?! I can eat in the classroom if I need to?!), but most of it was really terrifying. I really didn't like that I couldn't eat when I was hungry or that I had to eat when I wasn't. I was afraid of what would happen to me if I had a terrible low. I was afraid of what would happen if my blood sugar got too high.

I think many people who *don't* live with diabetes think that we get diagnosed with it, get used to it, and then are over it. My story, and the stories of many women with diabetes, is different.

After the initial diagnosis you do get a little used to it. Finger pricks no longer intimidate you. Giving yourself an injection becomes second nature. You learn to treat your body like a science lab and record pre-meal blood sugar levels. So, you figure it out a little bit, and then life changes and you need to learn something else. Just when you have that issue figured out, life changes again. It's a constant learning process. Diabetes as a teenager is different from diabetes as a pregnant woman. Diabetes in the mind of a child is much different than diabetes in the mind of an adult. My years in medical school were very difficult because I was learning in detail all of the things that could go wrong with diabetes, and it terrified me. To make it harder, I didn't have any friends with diabetes or know any other women who were living with the same fears and challenges.

My diabetes story is still being written. I've lived with my diabetes for 25 years now. I took diabetes with me to France when I studied abroad in college. I lugged it through medical school and my residency program. Diabetes came with me around the world in planes and helicopters when I was a racer on a popular endurance reality show, *The Amazing Race*. Diabetes walked down the aisle with me as I married a very supportive man. I can't even begin to imagine where else I will go with my diabetes in tow! The point is, diabetes is always there. No vacations. No days off. No breaks. As women with diabetes, we need to know how it will be a part of our lives, and what we can do to make sure we are living our best lives. I learn something new about diabetes every day, and much of the time it's from other women who have been where I am going. Diabetes is complicated. And it's very important to know not only how it affects us physically, but also how it affects us on an emotional and spiritual level.

I know for sure that there is no one way to figure it all out. However, I do believe that with the right tools, we can be prepared to figure out what needs to be done in every challenging situation.

SOUL-SEARCHING

What were your thoughts about diabetes prior to your diagnosis? Do you think about diabetes differently now that you have the diagnosis? What have you learned that has surprised you?

_____

_____

_____

_____

What was the hardest thing for you when you learned that you had diabetes?

_____

_____

_____

What helped you move past some of your initial fears? If you have fears, what are some ways you can help calm those fears?

_____

_____

_____

So let's start by going back to basics: What is diabetes, exactly? It's important to understand the entire spectrum of diabetes, including the different types, so that we can effectively educate and relate to others.

In medical terms, diabetes is a metabolic disease that results in elevated blood glucose levels. Put simply, diabetes is a chronic disease that results in high levels of sugar in the blood. Diabetes goes by several names: type 1 diabetes, type 2 diabetes, adult onset diabetes, juvenile onset diabetes, the sugars, sugar diabetes, gestational diabetes, insulin-dependent diabetes, non-insulin-dependent diabetes, and prediabetes.

There is some basic physiology that we should all understand. When you eat food, the body breaks down all of the carbohydrates into glucose (sugar) that enters your bloodstream by getting absorbed through your gastrointestinal tract. (Throughout this book, we will use "glucose" and "sugar" interchangeably.) In response, your pancreas—an organ behind your stomach—releases insulin. Insulin allows the sugar to move out of the bloodstream and into your cells where it can be used for energy. This sugar is the basic fuel for the cells of your body. When glucose builds up in the blood instead of going into cells, it is toxic for the

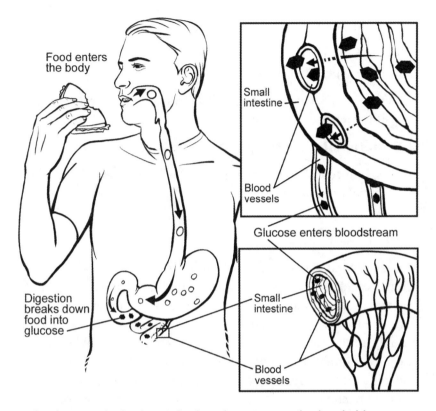

Food enters
the body

Small
intestine

Blood
vessels

Glucose enters bloodstream

Digestion
breaks down
food into
glucose

Small
intestine

Blood
vessels

As food enters the body, it is broken down into easily absorbable
components, including glucose. As glucose enters into the small intestine,
the small blood vessels take the glucose out of the gastrointestinal tract
and carry it into the bloodstream, to be delivered to your body for fuel.

body and can lead to health problems. Diabetes usually happens
because the body stops making insulin or because the body
becomes less responsive to insulin that is being made. Either way,
the insulin/glucose relationship is off balance, and the result is high
levels of sugar in the blood. It is also important to note that glucose
can be made in your body even if you are not eating any carbohydrates. Your liver has the ability to store and release sugar as your
body needs it. This is why there can be health problems due to low
insulin levels even if you are not eating at all.

Overall, there are four main types of diabetes:

- **Type 1 diabetes:** formerly called juvenile onset diabetes or insulin-dependent diabetes

- **Type 2 diabetes:** formerly called adult-onset diabetes or non-insulin-dependent diabetes

- **Gestational diabetes:** pregnancy diabetes

- **Prediabetes:** elevated blood sugar levels, but not high enough for a diabetes diagnosis

TYPE 1 DIABETES

This is the kind of diabetes that Brandy and I have. Type 1 diabetes often presents at a young age, but it is definitely possible for adults and even seniors to develop type 1 diabetes. My older brother was diagnosed with type 1 diabetes at age 36! Type 1 diabetes is an autoimmune disease that is caused by a combination of genetic and environmental triggers resulting in destruction of beta cells, and a lifelong dependency on the administration of insulin.

In plain English, due to a lot of influences, including our DNA and the world around us, the body loses its ability to make insulin. The body actually attacks and kills the insulin-producing cells in the pancreas. These insulin-making cells are called beta cells of the islets of Langerhans. Fancy name, right? When the beta cells are attacked and destroyed, the body doesn't have any way to make insulin and a lifelong dependency on insulin begins. Insulin is so important because this is the hormone that regulates carbohydrate, protein, and fat metabolism in the body. Insulin promotes uptake and use of the building blocks from dietary carbohydrate and fat for storage in our organs, as a source of future energy. Insulin promotes the uptake and retention of the building blocks of protein by our organs.

Furthermore, insulin prevents the breakdown of protein and prevents breakdown of storage forms of energy into fuels. Without insulin, energy from our food that should be stored in our bodies

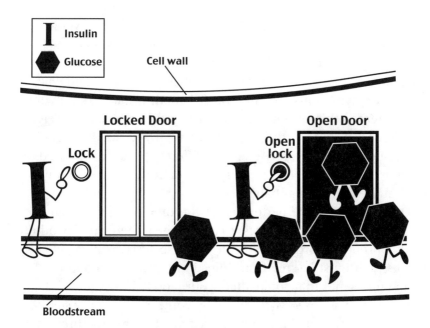

Without insulin, glucose has a hard time getting out of the bloodstream and to the organs that can use it for fuel. It's like trying to get through a locked door. Insulin acts like a key and opens the door so glucose can exit the bloodstream and get to the correct destination.

for later use is stuck in the bloodstream and not usable. As a result, our body breaks its own tissues down for energy. Uncontrolled diabetes in many ways resembles starvation.

Those of us living with type 1 diabetes have to take insulin, either by shots or insulin pumps, for survival. Without enough insulin, sugar will stay in the bloodstream where it is toxic, unusable, and can lead to devastating health problems. With too much insulin, hypoglycemia, or low blood sugar, can result. This can lead to mental changes, slowed thinking, shakiness, sweating, weakness, rapid heart rate, and even loss of consciousness. So, it's a constant balancing act to have enough insulin on board to get sugar into our cells, but not so much insulin that it takes too much sugar out of our bloodstream and leads to hypoglycemia (low blood sugar).

According to the Centers for Disease Control and Prevention's *National Diabetes Statistics Report, 2014,* 13.4 million women aged 20 years or older in the U.S. had diabetes in 2012. This number includes diagnosed and undiagnosed diabetes and type 1 and type 2. The classic symptoms are polyuria (frequent urination), polydipsia (increased thirst), polyphagia (increased hunger), and weight loss. Type 1 diabetes is diagnosed primarily by testing for elevated blood sugar levels. There are several different tests that are used to diagnose type 1 diabetes, and I will outline the most common ones at the end of this chapter.

Other tests may be performed at the time of type 1 diagnosis (such as thyroid function tests) to determine if there are any other health problems present. For all of these tests to give reliable results, you must be free from infections and viruses and not be taking medicines that could affect your blood glucose.

If you're diagnosed with diabetes, you may also be tested for autoantibodies that are common in type 1 diabetes (through a c-peptide test). These tests can help distinguish between type 1 and type 2 diabetes. The presence of ketones (byproducts from the breakdown of fat) in your urine also suggests type 1 diabetes, rather than type 2 diabetes.

Once you've been diagnosed with type 1 diabetes, you'll regularly visit your doctor to ensure good diabetes management. During these visits, the doctor will check your A1C levels. Your target A1C goal may vary depending on your age and various other factors, but the American Diabetes Association generally recommends that A1C levels be below 7%, which translates to an estimated average glucose of 154 mg/dl (8.5 mmol/l).

TYPE 2 DIABETES

Type 2 diabetes is by far the most common form of diabetes. According to the American Diabetes Association, 12.6 million, or roughly 11% of all women aged 20 years or older have type 2 diabetes. Unlike type 1 diabetes, in type 2 diabetes, the body is still able to make insulin. Diabetes develops with insulin in your system because either the body does not produce enough insulin or the cells in the body don't respond normally to insulin. When your fat, liver, and muscle cells do not respond correctly to insulin, this is called insulin resistance. As a result, blood sugar does not get out of the bloodstream and into your cells to be used or stored for energy. This is called hyperglycemia, or elevated blood sugar. Because increased fat in your body makes it harder to use insulin in the correct way, most people with the disease are overweight when they are diagnosed. Although being overweight increases the risk for type 2 diabetes, type 2 can also develop in people who are thin and/or who have a significant family history for diabetes.

Family history and genes play a large role in type 2 diabetes. Other risk factors include low activity level, poor diet, and excess body weight around your belly. Type 2 diabetes usually occurs slowly over time. Often, people with type 2 diabetes have no symptoms at first. They may not have symptoms for many years. This is why it is important to be screened for high blood sugar if you have a family history or risk factors.

Your health care provider may suspect that you have diabetes if your blood sugar level is ≥200 mg/dl, and the diagnosis is confirmed if there are classic symptoms of hyperglycemia or hyperglycemia crisis. Otherwise, to confirm the diagnosis, more tests need to be done. We will go over these tests below under "Diagnostic Tests for Diabetes."

THE SYMPTOMS OF TYPE 2 DIABETES MAY INCLUDE:

- increased thirst
- increased urination
- blurred vision
- bladder, kidney, skin, or other infections that are more frequent or that heal slowly
- sexual dysfunction
- pain or numbness in the feet or hands

Diabetes screening is recommended for:

- overweight children who have other risk factors for diabetes, starting at age 10 and repeated every 3 years

- overweight adults (body mass index [BMI] $\geq 25\,kg/m^2$) who have other risk factors

- adults aged 45 years or older every 3 years if results are normal. There should be consideration of more frequent testing if initial results suggest an elevated risk status

The goal of treatment at first is to lower high blood glucose levels to a safe range and to treat any side effects that are present at diagnosis. The long-term goals of treatment are to make lifestyle and medication changes to prevent problems from diabetes.

The treatment options for type 2 diabetes range widely depending on each individual's unique makeup, characteristics, and situation (blood glucose level, A1C level, other coexisting illnesses, etc.). Treatment may include diet, exercise, medications, injections, or any combination of the above. There is one common treatment that every woman with type 2 diabetes should adhere to, and that is optimizing diet and exercise. I know that this sounds simple, but diabetes is a metabolic condition, and needs metabolic attention. This means being very educated about what food goes into your mouth, and what your body does with that food. Everyone is different, and you should work closely with your health care provider to determine what dietary and exercise changes are best for you as an individual.

PREDIABETES

Prediabetes, also known as "impaired glucose tolerance" or "impaired fasting glucose," is a health condition with no symptoms. It is almost always present before a person develops the more serious type 2 diabetes. About 79 million people in the United States over the age of 20 have prediabetes, with blood sugar levels that are higher than normal, but are not high enough to be classified as diabetes. Without intervention, prediabetes is likely to become type 2 diabetes in 10 years or less.

More and more, doctors are recognizing the importance of diagnosing prediabetes, as treatment of the condition may prevent more serious health problems. Early diagnosis and treatment of prediabetes may prevent type 2 diabetes as well as associated complications such as heart and blood vessel disease and eye and kidney disease. Doctors now know that the health complications associated with type 2 diabetes often occur before the medical diagnosis of diabetes is made. In other words, far too many people are walking around with diabetes for many years before it is ever diagnosed.

There's good news, however. Prediabetes can be an opportunity for you to improve your health, because progression from prediabetes to type 2 diabetes isn't inevitable (25% of those with prediabetes develop diabetes within 3–5 years of diagnosis). With healthy lifestyle changes—such as eating healthy foods, including physical activity in your daily routine, and maintaining a healthy weight—you may be able to bring your blood sugar levels back to normal.

Here are strategies to decrease your risk of going from prediabetes to type 2 diabetes:

- Eat healthy meals that are low in fat, low in sugar, and low in salt.

- Exercise for 30 minutes a day at least 5 days a week as directed by your physician.

- Reduce your weight by as little as 5–10% if you are overweight, since this can have a significant impact on overall health.

GESTATIONAL DIABETES

Gestational diabetes develops during pregnancy. Like other types of diabetes, gestational diabetes affects how your cells use sugar (glucose)—your body's main fuel. Gestational diabetes causes high blood sugar that can affect your pregnancy and your baby's health.

Any pregnancy complication is concerning, but there's good news. Expectant moms can help control gestational diabetes by eating healthy foods, exercising and, if necessary, using medica-

In gestational diabetes, blood sugar usually returns to normal soon after delivery. But if you've had gestational diabetes, you're at risk for type 2 diabetes in the future. You'll want to continue working with your health care team to monitor and manage your blood sugar.

tion. Taking good care of yourself can ensure a healthy pregnancy for you and a healthy start for your baby.

Researchers don't yet know exactly why some women develop gestational diabetes. To understand how gestational diabetes occurs, it can help to understand how pregnancy affects your body's normal processing of glucose.

During all pregnancies, the placenta that connects your growing baby to your blood supply produces high levels of various hormones. Almost all of them impair the action of insulin in your cells, potentially raising your blood sugar. Modest elevation of blood sugar after meals is normal during pregnancy. However, it is when the action of insulin is impaired too much and blood sugar levels become too elevated that gestational diabetes is diagnosed.

As your baby grows, the placenta produces more insulin-blocking hormones. In gestational diabetes, the placental hormones provoke a rise in blood sugar to a level that can affect the growth and welfare of your baby. Gestational diabetes usually develops during the last half of pregnancy.

Medical experts haven't established a single set of screening guidelines for gestational diabetes, though this has been recognized as an area that needs attention for some time now. Many doctors now test all pregnant women for gestational diabetes at 26 weeks of gestation. However, the U.S. Preventive Services Task Force (USP-STF) recently concluded with moderate certainty that there is a moderate net benefit to screening for gestational diabetes after 24 weeks of gestation to reduce maternal and fetal complications (the collective outcomes of preeclampsia, macrosomia, and shoulder dystocia).

Your doctor will check your blood sugar after delivery and again in 6–12 weeks to make sure that your level has returned to normal. If your tests are normal—and most are—you'll need to have your diabetes risk assessed at least every 3 years. If your doctor does not order your blood sugar to be tested at least every 3 years, advocate for the blood glucose test yourself. The worst-case scenario is for you to be one of the millions of women walking around with undiagnosed diabetes. Knowledge is power. If future tests indicate diabetes or prediabetes, talk with your doctor about increasing your prevention efforts or starting a diabetes management plan.

DIAGNOSTIC TESTS FOR DIABETES

Fasting Blood Glucose (FBG)

In a FBG test, a blood sample is obtained after a period of fasting for at least 8 hours. This usually means no food or drink (except water) is taken after midnight on the night before the test. A blood sample is usually drawn early the next day before any food is eaten or beverages consumed. If the results of this test reveal a glucose reading of 126 mg/dl or higher it indicates diabetes. To confirm the diagnosis, it is usually necessary to repeat the test a second time on a different day. Fasting glucose levels are normally between 70 and 100 mg/dl in a person without diabetes. The FBG test is the most commonly used test for diagnosing diabetes in general.

Random Blood Glucose

In a random blood glucose test, a blood sample is also tested to measure your glucose but there is no consideration given to when you ate your last meal. A glucose level greater than or equal to 200 mg/dl indicates that you have diabetes if you also have other symptoms like increased thirst, increased hunger, or increased urination. This is the preferred glucose test used in medical emergencies when a person (most often a child) has such high blood sugar levels they may be drifting into a diabetes-induced coma. Within minutes of using this test, medical personnel can determine how much glucose is in the blood and administer insulin if type 1 diabetes is confirmed as the diagnosis.

Oral Glucose Tolerance Test (OGTT)

This diagnostic test, called the oral glucose tolerance test, differs from the other two because you are asked to drink a sugary beverage as a way to measure how your pancreas can manage the glucose you take in. Before you drink the beverage, a baseline fasting blood glucose is taken. You then drink the beverage and over the next 2 hours blood glucose levels are taken every 30 minutes. In a person without diabetes, glucose levels rise and then fall quickly because the body naturally produces insulin to lower the blood glucose. In contrast, a person with type 1 diabetes will see a sharp rise and a sustained high level of glucose because the pancreas is unable to deliver the needed insulin to lower the glucose in the blood. This test is often administered to pregnant women during the third trimester to test for gestational diabetes.

If your blood glucose at the 2-hour mark is below 140 mg/dl, your blood sugar is considered normal. If the reading is between 141 and 199 mg/dl, prediabetes is indicated. A reading that exceeds or is equal to 200 mg/dl after the same time period indicates diabetes. If glucose levels are higher than or equal to 200 mg/dl, the test should be repeated on a different day to confirm the diagnosis.

Understanding the OGTT Test Results	
Condition	OGTT at 2 hours
Normal	<140 mg/dl
Prediabetes	140 mg/dl to 199 mg/dl
Diabetes	≥200 mg/dl

A1C (hemoglobin A1C) test

The hemoglobin A1C test has traditionally been a measure of long-term control of glucose levels in the bloodstream. But in 2010, the American Diabetes Association recommended that the test also be used as another option for diagnosing diabetes and prediabetes. Though using the A1C test would more often be used for diagnosing type 2 diabetes, it deserves mention here because it could also be used to diagnose type 1.

When glucose test results on the A1C measure 6.5% or higher on blood hemoglobin, it is considered a diagnosis for diabetes. The advantages of using the A1C test over plasma glucose is that it takes less time and is more convenient than the oral glucose tolerance test and does not require fasting before the test is performed.

DIABETES BLOOD TESTS

- **Fasting Blood Glucose Level:** Diabetes is diagnosed if it is higher than 126 mg/dl, two times. (If your blood glucose at the 2-hour mark is below 140 mg/dl, your blood sugar is considered normal. A reading that is ≥200 mg/dl after the same time period indicates diabetes. If glucose levels are ≥200 mg/dl, the test should be repeated on a different day to confirm the diagnosis.)

- **Hemoglobin A1C Test**
  Normal: Less than 5.7%
  Prediabetes: 5.7% to 6.4%
  Diabetes: 6.5% or higher

- **Oral Glucose Tolerance Test:** Diabetes is diagnosed if glucose level is higher than 200 mg/dl after 2 hours.

PREDIABETES BLOOD TESTS

- Fasting blood glucose level of 100–125 mg/dl (5.6–6.9 mmol/l)
- A 2-hour glucose tolerance test after ingesting the standardized 75-gram glucose solution shows a blood sugar level of 140–199 mg/dl (7.8–11.0 mmol/l)

- Hemoglobin A1C of between 5.7% and 6.4%

A1C EQUIVALENTS TO AVERAGE BLOOD SUGAR LEVELS

A1C percentage	mg/dl	mmol/l
6%	126	7.0
6.5%	140	7.8
7%	154	8.6
7.5%	169	9.4
8%	183	10.1
8.5%	197	10.9
9%	212	11.9
9.5%	226	12.6
10%	240	13.4

Other tests may be performed at the time of diagnosis (such as thyroid) to determine if there are any other autoimmune antibodies present. For all of these tests to give reliable results, you must be free from infections and viruses and not be taking medicines that could affect your blood glucose.

SOUL-SEARCHING

What kind of diabetes do you have?

_____

What are some things you can do to improve your health?

_____

What was your most recent A1C level?

_____

What is your goal A1C level?

_____

Have you, along with your health care team, discussed a plan for getting you to that A1C level?

_____

If so, what is your plan?

_____

_____

_____

_____

_____

If not, what initiative can you take to "get the ball rolling" with your health care team? (Or is it time to create your diabetes health care team?)

_____

_____

_____

_____

_____

Now that we have gone over the physiology of diabetes, and the way it is diagnosed, it's time to think about what diabetes means to you. Understanding what diabetes is, and how it works, is important so that you can understand what does and doesn't affect your diabetes. I encourage you to use this chapter as a basis for understanding and applying everything else in this book. Diabetes is big. It's dynamic. It's complicated. What seems to work one day may not the next, and it's important to make sure your knowledge base is continuously growing so that you can keep up! I've had diabetes for over 25 years, and I am still learning new things!

🔘 LIFE APPLICATION

Test your knowledge! Take this true/false test, then check out the answers below.

1. The type of diabetes a woman has is based on how old she was when she was diagnosed.

2. If I am taking insulin, it means that I have type 1 diabetes.

3. You can tell what type of diabetes a woman has by whether or not she is overweight. If she is overweight, she has type 2 diabetes.

4. Having gestational diabetes puts me at higher risk for developing type 2 diabetes later on.

5. Overweight children who have a family history of diabetes should be screened every 2 years starting at age 15.

Answers:

1. *False.* Type 2 diabetes can develop in children, and type 1 diabetes can develop in adults. Sometimes it is not clear at first what kind of diabetes you have. I have heard several stories of women who were wrongly classified as having type 2 diabetes because they were adults at the time of diagnosis. Make sure to be your own best advocate with your doctor. If you aren't seeing good results with your diabetes care despite following your doctor's recommendations, consider asking for further testing or an appointment with a specialist to get the correct diagnosis.

2. *False.* While it is true that every person with type 1 diabetes will need to take insulin, some people with type 2 diabetes will also need to take insulin. Likewise, some of the traditional type 2 med-

ications are now being used in the care of type 1 diabetes. The best way to know what kind of diabetes you have is to have a C-peptide test performed at a lab.

3. *False.* You cannot tell what type of diabetes a person has based solely on her weight. Being overweight is a risk factor for type 2 diabetes, but there are overweight women with type 1 diabetes, too.

4. *True.* Having gestational diabetes can put you at a higher risk for type 2 diabetes later in life. It's important to be aware of steps that you can take to prevent or delay this. Make sure you keep up on the recommended screening guidelines.

5. *False.* Overweight children who have other risk factors for diabetes (like a family history) should be screened every 3 years starting at age 10.

NOTES ON MY JOURNEY

_____

_____

_____

_____

_____

_____

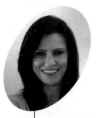

Mental Wellness

BRANDY SAYS...

The date was Monday, January 21, 1991, and I was a high school sophomore in Hickory, North Carolina. My mom and I were awaiting the results from my blood and urine tests at the pediatrician's office. I glanced out the window into the peaceful courtyard and thought about how just the night before, after taking note of how much water I was drinking, my mom nervously suggested that she make a doctor's appointment for me. After hearing her and my dad whispering in their bedroom, I asked, "What is it? What do you think I have? Why do I need to go to the doctor?" With a bit of hesitation, my mom said, "Well, you know your dad's sister, JoAnn, has diabetes. We just want to make sure that you don't have it too."

I spent the rest of that Sunday evening researching the disease called diabetes that I knew very little about. As soon as I read the symptoms (excessive thirst, lethargy, blurred vision, and frequent urination), my heart sank, because they all fit me. I called a few friends and frantically told them that I thought I had diabetes. They reassured me that I didn't.

Now as my mom and I sat in the exam room awaiting the results, I began to contemplate the impact of being diagnosed with this disease: It was the middle of basketball season and I was a starting player on the JV basketball team. Will diabetes eliminate me from the team? What about my friends? Will they act differently toward me? Will I still be able to go to the college I've always dreamed of, the University of North Carolina (UNC) at Chapel Hill? And what about my dream of traveling the world as an investigative journalist? How would diabetes fit into that grand plan? Until then, I had been living a pretty normal teenage life, playing sports, serving on the high school newspaper staff, and taking the classes I needed to get into UNC Chapel Hill.

Then the nurse walked into the room with a smile on her face and said, "Everything came back fine. You're free to go!" And she left. My mom and I breathed a sigh of relief and stood up to leave.

Then the door opened again, and the doctor walked in looking very distraught. "I'm sorry," he said. "The nurse made a mistake. She read the wrong results. You *do* have diabetes and you need to go straight to the hospital." He told us that my blood sugar was 450mg/dl, a dangerously high level. I don't really know what else he said because I had escaped into my own head and began to think, "They must have made a mistake again. It can't be true! I *know* I don't have diabetes! They *just* told me I didn't have diabetes!"

Denial was rearing its ugly head. Denial is a powerful tool that many of us employ during the early stages of diabetes. I had to face my diagnosis while in the midst of my teen angst, but it's hard to face no matter how old you are. For me, the denial stage was relatively short-lived, lasting through the first day and a half of my week-long hospital stay. (Yes, that tells you how long ago I was diagnosed because I actually stayed in the hospital for a week!) Your stint(s) in the denial phase may be much shorter or longer. Everyone is different.

THE ROAD TO ACCEPTANCE

The road to acceptance is usually littered with puddles (okay, sometimes flood waters) of grief. This is not terribly surprising. After all, we are mourning life as we knew it: Life without disease. Life without restrictions. Life with a working pancreas. A carefree life that was often taken for granted.

Over the years, a number of people have offered theories and suggestions about how to get through a diabetes diagnosis. In 1969, psychiatrist Elisabeth Kübler-Ross introduced what became known as the "five stages of grief." They are denial, anger, bargaining, depression, and acceptance. Contrary to popular belief, you do not have to go through each stage in order to heal. You probably won't experience these stages in a neat, sequential order, so don't worry about what you "should" be feeling or which stage you're supposed to be in.

In fact, Kübler-Ross never intended for these stages to be a rigid framework that applies to everyone who mourns. In her last book before her death in 2004, she said of the five stages of grief: "They were never meant to help tuck messy emotions into neat packages. They are responses to loss that many people have, but *there is not a typical response to loss, as there is no typical loss.* Our grieving is as individual as our lives."

I have also heard some compare post-diagnosis grief to a roller coaster ride: The peaks and valleys are much more intense at first, but they become shorter and less intense over time. Grieving is a natural and highly individual experience. However you choose to look at them, there are some common experiences and feelings that are felt by most women post-diagnosis. Let's take a look at what these stages look like in women with diabetes.

In addition to Kübler-Ross' five stages, I am also proposing a sixth stage that is often seen in women with diabetes: Guilt.

THE SIX STAGES OF DIABETES GRIEF

Denial

Shock and disbelief are common when someone is diagnosed with diabetes. "There must be a mistake." Most often, denial is displayed when a person tries to continue life as "normal"—as if the diagnosis never occurred. I expressed denial by temporarily shutting down and isolating myself. This was my way of avoiding the diagnosis. I slept a lot, and if I wasn't sleeping, I was staring at the hospital wall. I recall hearing my mom talking to a nurse outside the door to my room, and saying, "I'm really worried about her." This was probably a mixture of denial and depression. As I mentioned, the stages don't always happen in sequential order or in a pretty package with a tag that reads, "Welcome to the 'denial' stage." It's up to you to identify which stage(s) you are in based on your own thoughts and behaviors.

Fear of the unknown is a major part of this stage, and that's easy to understand. There is so much "unknown" after a diabetes diagnosis. It could be compared to finding out you are pregnant. (Although, hopefully, you are much happier when you get this news!) In both situations, you know that your life is about to change in some major ways, but you just have to live through it to understand and appreciate it.

The resounding theme I hear from women with diabetes is that they feel "defective." It is incredibly difficult for many women to accept that their body has let them down. Having a pancreas that doesn't work properly or doesn't work at all means that the body is no longer working at 100%, no longer in tip-top shape. Anything less than 100% is defective, and defective is far from the perfection that is depicted on the cover of magazines and in television shows.

It's easier to believe that nothing has changed. The human mind is a very protective organ. Before jumping head-first into a major lifestyle change, the human brain takes us each on a unique journey during which we gradually work through the enormity of such a diagnosis. While everyone does not go through every stage, no one walks out of the doctor's office on that first day in the acceptance stage.

A woman in the denial stage may say things like, "I only have a touch of diabetes," or, "The doctor didn't say I had diabetes, he just said my blood sugar was a little high." Or she might not say anything at all because she thinks that if she doesn't talk about it, it doesn't exist. I recall one woman who shared with me how she kept avoiding returning to the doctor, saying, "As long as I don't hear the words, 'You have diabetes,' I don't have it." Eventually, the doctor sent her a letter via certified mail, so although she avoided hearing the words, she eventually had to read them in black and white. She told me that in hindsight, she would have rather heard those life-changing words from a human being than reading them alone in her living room.

The important thing to understand is that the diabetes diagnosis will catch up with you, maybe not today, but one day. Then you may wish you had acknowledged reality sooner so that you could have prevented complications. For the most part, a woman in denial makes few, if any, of the lifestyle changes that diabetes requires. She may refuse to take medications, check her blood sugar, change her diet, or exercise regularly. As a result, complications develop more rapidly because her blood sugar is out of control. Uncontrolled blood sugars can lead to the early onset of retinopathy (eye disease) and vision loss, nephropathy (kidney disease) and dialysis, neuropathy (nerve disease) and amputations, cardiovascular disease (heart disease), heart attacks, and can lead to an early death. Where's the good news in this?

As my good friend and colleague Bill Polonsky often says, "Well-controlled diabetes is the leading cause of . . . nothing!" In other words, gaining control of your diabetes early has some pretty nice rewards; No (or at least fewer) diabetes complications. If you are in the denial phase, friends may try to "snap you out of it," assume you need more diabetes education, or accuse you of being illogical. In reality, you are the only one who can help yourself out of this stage. If you feel you are stuck in the denial stage, contact a mental health professional, attend a peer diabetes support group, and/or reach out to someone via an online diabetes community.

Anger

"Ducking Fiabetes!" "I hate this disease!" "It's not fair!" "Why me?" Anger can range from minor frustration to full-blown rage. In its most severe form, anger can be all-consuming and destructive, ruining marriages and wiping out families. The problem with anger is that it never just affects the newly diagnosed. Loved ones (nearest and dearest) often experience the brunt of the anger.

You have probably observed a few people in the anger stage. The first thing you notice about them is how unhappy they are. Being angry can really isolate you. It is a vicious cycle: You are mad at the world about your diabetes, and this anger makes you unattractive and unapproachable to friends and potential mates. Then you blame the fact that you have few friends/love interests on the fact that you have diabetes and the disease makes you "less than." You continue to be mad at the world because your diabetes is making your friends avoid you. The world sees you as unapproachable and unattractive because you are so angry.

Anger about diabetes   Small support network

If you are on this merry-go-round, the best way to get off is to turn your anger to more positive activities and focus on things you can do something about. In reality, persistent anger is just a waste of your precious time. Instead, think about how you could direct that energy into a focused action that would make a positive impact on diabetes for you and everyone else with diabetes. For example, if you feel like no one understands how hard it is to have diabetes, try educating others about what a day is like in the life of a person with diabetes. Try using your unique skills and attributes (one of which is diabetes) to take what you see as a negative and turn it into a positive.

Although it is hard to believe sometimes, diabetes *is* a unique attribute and something that makes you interesting to many other people. How *you* choose to view *your* diabetes affects the way everyone with whom you come

"Comparison is the thief of joy."

Theodore Roosevelt

into contact with views it. In today's world, everybody is trying to figure out what their unique quality is so that they can stand out from the crowd. You don't have to look far to find your unique quality. You just have to think about how to present the unique quality of diabetes in a positive, flattering way.

For example, instead of talking about diabetes as an inconvenience, you can talk about all you have accomplished while living with diabetes. If you talk about the fact that diabetes is only a small part of who you are, those around you will receive a very different message about diabetes and about *you*. As talk show therapist Dr. Phil says: "You teach people how to treat you." Do you celebrate your unique characteristic (diabetes) and "OWN" it or do you apologetically tuck your diabetes away in a drawer hoping no one sees your weakness? We'll come back to this idea of "OWNing" your diabetes later.

Sometimes, the diabetes diagnosis becomes very personal for those in the anger stage, as though someone or something has fulfilled a grudge against them. They are mad at the world because they have a disease and no one else around them does. As a result, they become very critical. Through the DiabetesSisters' Conference Series, PODS (Part of DiabetesSisters) support groups, and various other in-person events, I have seen the anger stage manifested in a number of different ways.

During my time at the helm of DiabetesSisters, I have come into contact with thousands of women with diabetes. My staff and I have learned to detect those in the anger stage; their anger is very much at the surface and it is voiced not just once, but many times about many different things. We can tell someone is in this stage because the *level* of her anger does not seem appropriate to the situation. For example, a woman may be enraged that topics weren't discussed *in the way* she wanted, or that we discussed topics she *did not* want to discuss. She may be livid that we ran out of fruit at lunch or that her husband wasn't allowed to attend a conference session with her. What she says she is angry about is not really the source of her anger. Her diabetes is usually the source, and this should be taken into consideration when working with her.

Some of these women return year after year, and our team gracefully listens to their complaints. But the best-case scenarios are those women who, over time, move beyond the anger stage into well-adjusted, successful women with diabetes. What a joy to see—and be around!

Self-pity is another common component of the anger stage. Someone experiencing self-pity might ask, "Why me?" But she might also compare herself to those who do not have diabetes. This comparison leads to a feeling that this misfortune should have happened to someone else. You may think that someone with many more perceived faults is more deserving of a diabetes diagnosis. To outsiders, those who are experiencing self-pity appear to feel as though they have been "done wrong" and/or that the world owes them something.

It is not uncommon for ongoing thoughts of self-pity to develop into a long-term victim mentality. Being a victim is as much about one's own perception as reality, if not more. If you are alive and breathing, you have had something bad happen to you in life. Every woman has been taken advantage of, duped, betrayed, or treated unfairly at some point in her life. If you focus on acts of betrayal or negative things that have happened to you, they will take over your life. Victims have a sad story to tell and tell it often to whomever will listen. In many different life situations, victims feel persecuted or abused in some way. A victim may be deeply hurt by the cab driver who made an unkind comment about people with diabetes, or wounded by the friend who did not appropriately acknowledge how hard her life (with diabetes) really is.

Victims are the women we feel sorry for. They usually have a lot of drama in their lives and may even be referred to as "drama queens" by their friends and family. The truth is that they make us appreciate how uncomplicated our own lives are. I have seen many women get stuck in the victim mentality, who have surrounded themselves with an entire support team who "buy into" their victimization.

If you are stuck in the victim mentality, you likely have a spouse/significant other, friends, family, and/or co-workers who go out of their way to make sure you are comfortable and happy because of this disease that was unfairly thrust upon you. These are your "enablers." It can be hard to recognize enablers because they are so full of love and admiration for you. They genuinely love you and want you to be happy in life. Unfortunately, your happiness has taken precedence over their happiness and this has permanently changed the balance of power in your household to benefit you. As harsh as it may sound, you have become a "taker."

Although they are receiving a lot from others (help, support, etc.), the victim is the one who is paying the ultimate price. Your personal growth is stunted by those who buy in to your victimization, so you have very little chance of growing or of reaching your full potential in life. You may even become complacent in this kind of mentality because it's hard to give up the comforts of being on this kind of "victim pedestal." Willingly stepping out on a limb to a life where work is required and success is earned is very scary. There is fear of the unknown, fear of failure, and the knowledge that once you step out of the victim mentality and others see a glimpse of how strong you really are, there's no going back.

If you think you might be stuck in the victim mentality, you probably are. If you're wondering whether or not it is worth it to move out of the victim mentality, consider this: Although it is not easy to change, it *is* possible with consistent work. Remember, nothing worth having in life comes easily. It takes a strong woman to admit this and make the change, but you already know you are a strong woman because you have lived with diabetes. Furthermore, the fact that you are reading this book suggests that you are open to change and want to try new ideas to improve your life with diabetes. The change must start in your mind. A person or situation can only hurt or victimize you if you allow it to do so. You are, and always will be, in control of your perspective.

A woman with diabetes who is in the anger stage might not be easy to help. She is on the defensive and she puts those around her on the defensive. However, the best thing you can give her is support and understanding. Counseling and peer support groups offer the best help for a woman who is stuck in the anger stage

> "For every minute you are angry, you lose 60 seconds of happiness."
>
> *Ralph Waldo Emerson*

because they provide a safe place for her to vent about and work through her emotional issues. There is little time for such counseling during doctor visits.

If you are a woman who is in the anger phase, you can take an important step by simply acknowledging that you are, indeed, angry about your diabetes. That is the first big hurdle. The next part of working through your anger is to ask yourself, "What am I really angry about?" This is where pen and paper are the most useful. This may take a lot of soul-searching, but it is well worth the time and effort when you begin to see your anger dissipate and your life become more enjoyable.

Bargaining

When a woman thinks she can control some uncontrollable aspect of diabetes through her short-term behavior, she is in the bargaining stage. Bargaining keeps her from accepting something that she doesn't want to accept.

If you recently said or thought something like "God, please, if you take away my diabetes, I promise I will never [insert negative habit with which you struggle] again," or, "Please, if you let me have a good checkup with the eye doctor today, I won't eat [insert your favorite unhealthy food here] for the next 2 weeks," you are in the bargaining phase. Generally, bargaining includes the phrase "If . . . , then . . . ," and it includes unrealistic outcomes (taking away diabetes or having a glowing report from the doctor despite negative health behaviors).

Sometimes people in the bargaining stage turn to alternative therapies and experimental drugs. In the diabetes world, there seems to be a new radical "cure" for diabetes every week, everything from cinnamon to magic pills. Unfortunately, a lot of people take advantage of people with diabetes who are stuck in the vulnerable bargaining phase.

If you recognize that you are in the bargaining phase, you can start by patting yourself on the back. Acknowledgment is the first step toward moving out of this stage. Now it is time to accept the fact that your reality is just not going to change. No matter how hard you try or how much you bargain with a higher power, your diabetes is not going away. (Note: Even if you have type 2 diabetes and are able to make healthy lifestyle changes that allow you come off of insulin or stop taking diabetes medications, diabetes will always be lurking under the surface. It never goes away.)

Once you've accepted this, you can make a decision to stop trying to fight against your diagnosis and, instead, work *with* your diagnosis. It's important to identify something to replace this coping mechanism. Each time you start to have an "if. . .then. . ." thought related to your diabetes, replace the thought with a healthy behavior, like checking your blood sugar or researching new forms of fun exercise for you and your best friend to try out. Repetition is the way we learn to create a new habit; research shows that it takes 21 days to form a new habit.

Depression

While rates of depression among people with diabetes are nearly double those of their nondiabetic peers, being a woman with diabetes further increases that risk. When you think about it, it makes perfect sense. People with diabetes have a lot to deal with on a daily basis. In fact, behavioral researcher Kate Lorig once attempted to count the number of things a person with diabetes must do on a daily basis. She stopped counting at 150! That's 150 tasks on top of all of the other daily requirements of life. Add to that the dynamic role that women play in families and you begin to think, "It's *no surprise* that depression is such a big issue for women with diabetes!"

The severity of depression in people with diabetes is often unacknowledged, especially in the medical field. There are a number of reasons that the health care team may not acknowledge or ask about depression during a visit. The first reason is simply lack of time during the alloted 15-minute visit. The second reason is due to a lack of resources. Physicians pride themselves on finding solutions to people's health problems. However, there are very few mental health professionals who specialize in diabetes-related depression. This puts a lot of responsibility into the hands of the person with diabetes to identify his or her own depression and find resources for treatment. While it is a very serious condition, being depressed does not mean that you are weak-minded. It can be overcome, if addressed properly.

So how do you know if you are just a little sad or if you are clinically depressed? This is one of the most commonly asked questions among our conference attendees. According to the DSM-IV (which is the document used by the American Psychiatric Association to identify mental health disorders), if you have *five or more* of the following symptoms for a period of at least 2 weeks and they interfere with your ability to perform the daily activities, you should seek the help of a mental health professional.

- Sadness, irritability, or "empty" mood that lasts most of the day, nearly every day
- A loss of pleasure or interest in doing things you used to enjoy
- Feelings of hopelessness or pessimism
- Decreased energy, fatigue, and feeling "slowed down"
- Difficulty concentrating, remembering, and making decisions
- Feelings of worthlessness, inappropriate guilt, or helplessness
- Insomnia, early-morning awakening, or oversleeping
- Changes in appetite; eating either more or less than you used to (when not dieting), resulting in changes in weight
- Nervousness or restlessness
- Recurrent thoughts of death (should be differentiated from a fear of dying) or suicidal thoughts

You may have any combination of these symptoms and some may be more severe than others. The biggest difference between sadness and depression is the length of time you experience the symptoms. If it has only been a few days or a week, it is sadness. If it has lasted for at least the last 2 weeks, you should seek the help of a mental health professional because it is likely depression. Also, if you observe a recurring pattern in your sadness (maybe it comes for a few days, then goes for a few days, then comes back for a few days), you should seek the help of a mental health professional.

There are a number of different types of depression, including major depression, chronic depression (dysthymia), and bipolar disorder. Some are more debilitating than others. Keep in mind that the most commonly reported symptom of depression is a loss of interest in things that you previously enjoyed. Depression is *not* something that can be willed or wished away. It affects the way you look at the world and how you feel about yourself. Sadly, some women live with chronic depression and never seek treatment, which dulls their chances of living a happy, healthy life with diabetes. Even more heartbreaking are the women with the more severe type of depression (major depression), who take their own lives because they see no other way out. I want to be very clear that depression is a very serious disorder and should be given proper consideration, particularly among women with diabetes—who are at an increased risk.

Loss of control is often a contributing factor to depression in women with diabetes. Women tend to be "in control" of a lot of activities in their lives and in the lives of their family members. A disease like diabetes throws that sense of control into a complete tailspin. Like an uninvited houseguest, diabetes just appeared in your life one day out of nowhere—without calling ahead. The unwanted houseguest shows up with way too much luggage, never cleans up after herself, and expects to be the center of attention at all times. And you have no way of evicting the guest, so she is destined to stay at your house for the rest of your life. No wonder diabetes is so exhausting for women!

One way diabetes differs from other life challenges is that no matter how hard you work or how well you organize your life, you do not have the power to make your diabetes go away. It is not like a debt that can be paid off. It is not like the extra baby weight that can be lost if you follow the right plan. You had no control over whether or not diabetes would enter your life, when it would enter your life, or how long it stays in your life.

If you are a women with a Type A personality, it would not be surprising to hear that your diabetes diagnosis was mentally crippling. This loss of control can make the whole world look different, and even a bit scary, because you may be fearful of the next life-altering illness or circumstance that will drop into your life.

Let's not forget what the average woman has to do on a daily basis, beyond the requirements of her diabetes. Many women still bear much of the responsibility for managing their households; they handle most of the domestic chores, plan social activities, manage finances, transport children to doctor appointments and extracurricular events, and handle the shopping, among other things.

On top of all this, many women are busy managing their careers. Having this kind of power can be both liberating and stressful. When is there any time left for a woman with diabetes to manage her own chronic illness (remember those 150+ daily diabetes tasks discussed earlier?) or tend to her own well-being?

If you are currently experiencing major depression and feeling hopeless, it is best to start with small steps. Just getting out of bed is a good first step. Taking a shower, getting dressed, and going outside the house are all positive steps. If you can take it one step further and engage in some physical activity, you have taken another important step toward moving beyond the depression stage. Breaking each goal into small steps and celebrating each one is important. Start looking for small subtle signs that things are getting better—like music sounding better, food tasting better, and colors looking brighter.

If you still feel stuck, keep in mind that depression is a serious illness, and focusing on a goal to get you through it may not be enough. No matter what kind of depression you are dealing with, treatment frequently requires medication and/or counseling from qualified mental health experts. They can help you rekindle the motivation you need to break through to the next stage.

Guilt

Wait! Before you skip this section because guilt is such a sensitive subject, I ask that you just hang in for a few more paragraphs. I think you will feel more understood and less guilty by the end of this section.

Guilt is a topic that often leaves that uncomfortable lump in your throat or pit in your stomach. We've all felt it at some point in our lives when we felt like we had done something wrong. For example, you may feel guilt when you make a hurtful comment or when you don't make it to your child's important game.

For women with type 1 and type 2 diabetes, numbers are often a source of guilt. Blood sugar readings, A1C levels, and weight are often used to gauge how well you are managing your diabetes. Your health care team congratulates or reprimands you based on these numbers. A high blood number translates into, "You did that to yourself. It's your fault." For many, this also translates into whether you are a "good" or "bad" person.

Making food choices can also lead to guilt. Eating healthy 100% of the time is difficult, if not impossible. Yet when we don't eat perfectly, we tell ourselves: "You shouldn't be eating that. You know it's going to mess up your blood sugar level. You are such a bad diabetic." It's important to realize that no one is perfect in managing diabetes, and that everyone is allowed—and even encouraged—to consume some fats and carbs every day. In fact, the American Diabetes Association recommends that adults with diabetes consume about 45 to 60 grams of carbohydrate per meal, which adds up to 135 to 180 grams of carbohydrates per day. Fat is also an important part of your diet. The American Heart Association currently recommends that 30% of your total caloric intake should come from fats. Fats will keep you from getting hungry between meals. Some women with diabetes go too far down the path of perfection and restriction when chasing good diabetes control.

Diabetes guilt is also rampant in the diabetes community because of the judgment of friends, family, coworkers, and society as a whole. Let's face it—society's blame is a huge burden to carry. This blame and shame often comes from incorrect, misleading, or incomplete information about the complex disease.

"And now that you don't have to be perfect, you can be good."

John Steinbeck

For many Americans, the only diabetes education has come from media outlets. Headlines scream "Diabetes Epidemic in U.S. Because Americans Eat Too Much," and, "Sedentary Lifestyle of American Kids Leads to Diabetes Epidemic." These kinds of headlines convey a really incomplete story when it comes to diabetes.

The headlines do not recognize that there is a strong genetic component to type 2 diabetes. As a result, women with diabetes (regardless of the type) who are overweight are particularly stigmatized by society. Many women choose not to share their diabetes diagnosis to avoid the looks of blame and disgust from strangers and loved ones.

This happens even in the most surprising places. I recently heard about a woman who was diagnosed with type 2 diabetes while working for one of the world's leading diabetes organizations. She chose not to tell her coworkers out of fear of their judgment. "You work at a diabetes organization with access to all of the latest preventive information. You should have taken better care of yourself!" These were the words she most feared. And that leads us to another difficult subject: the topic of blame and shame among women with different types of diabetes.

When I first starting getting active in the diabetes community in 2008, the thing that shocked me the most was the number of highly educated people who have an "elitist" mentality about their type of diabetes. "My diabetes is worse/better than yours," they would say, or, "My diabetes is nothing like your diabetes." All of these statements are filled with judgment and likely come from misdirected anger about one's own diabetes.

I have observed this elitist attitude much more often among women with type 1 diabetes than among those with type 2 diabetes; there is this desire to separate themselves from the bad publicity associated with type 2 diabetes. Some even want to change the names of the diseases (type 1 and type 2) so that there is less confusion about what they are and what they mean.

From my perspective, there are so many more important and positive battles that we could be fighting as a united community. It saddens me to say that, on occasion, I have even received angry emails from women with type 1 diabetes who mistakenly registered for the Weekend for Women conference believing that it was a type 1–only conference. Some have even refused to attend if there were going to be women with type 2 in attendance.

In my opening remarks at these conferences, I have encouraged women to open their minds and hearts to every woman in attendance regardless of age, race, home state, sexual orientation, or type of diabetes. There is so much to learn from someone who has a different perspective from you. But you have to open your mind (and let go of the guilt and shame) to be able to accept it.

At the conclusion of each conference, we ask women to rate their ability to support and receive support from women with other types of diabetes. To date, 96% of conference attendees agree or strongly agree that women with diabetes can effectively support and receive support from women with other types of diabetes. I know women with type 2 diabetes who became empowered to go on insulin after talking to women with type 1 who had been taking insulin for years. I have seen women with type 1 diabetes share everything from recipes to jewelry with women who have type 2 diabetes.

As women, we are our own best advocates. The best action we can take is to support our fellow sisters with diabetes, regardless of the type. After all, we have a much stronger voice when we all stand in unity than when we waste time bickering and competing among ourselves.

Misguided health professionals can also be sources of blame, shame, and guilt, saying things like, "If you would have gotten yourself together sooner, you could have prevented this from happening." Women walk away from these appointments feeling more responsible than ever that they caused the disease.

Women experiencing diabetes guilt often say the following to themselves: "If I'd taken better care, this would not have happened," or "I have diabetes because I am a bad person." This kind of negative talk wears on you over time and can lead to depression. If you have found yourself saying any of the above statements, now is the time to commit to stopping the "self-blame" and "self-hatred." Carrying around this kind of shame and guilt prevents you from reaching the ultimate goal of acceptance with diabetes. You did *not* cause this disease, so erase that statement from your head completely. Realize that you can only control what YOU can control, including such things as your perspective and your food choices. You cannot control others' perspectives or actions. Do the best you can do with the resources you have, and let God take care of those who want to inject negativity into your life. You have a lot to accomplish in this lifetime, right? Why waste any more time feeling undue guilt and shame?

Acceptance

Reaching the acceptance stage involves more than simply acknowledging that you have the disease. It's being able to finally say, "I have diabetes, and I'm okay with that." It is coming to terms with and making peace with the fact that you will have this chronic illness every day for the rest of your life and that you have to make unexpected alterations in your life to allow you to live a happy, healthy, productive life.

The majority of the women I know who have reached the acceptance stage have gotten there by finding purpose in their diagnosis. For some, the diabetes diagnosis was a wake-up call to live healthier lives, and to therefore be around longer to enjoy their grandchildren. For others, their diagnosis led to an entirely new career path for them. There is no limit to the purpose of your diabetes.

You'll know you have reached the acceptance stage when:

- you are at *peace* with the fact that you have diabetes and there's nothing you can do to change your diagnosis.

- you feel a sense of *freedom* and *gratitude* that you have the opportunity to shape your own future through your outlook and perspective.

- you feel a sense of *control* over diabetes. (That does not mean that you have a perfect A1C or perfect blood sugar readings.)

- you see diabetes as just another part of your daily life, like brushing your teeth.

Letting go of what you cannot control (being diagnosed with diabetes) and finding value in what you *can* control (blood sugar levels and mental outlook) are often key factors in acceptance of diabetes. Some women even reach the stage of acceptance where there is no regret. When asked whether they wish they had never been diagnosed with diabetes, they might say, "No, diabetes is a part of who I am. It has served a purpose in my life." If that seems far-fetched to you, don't worry: You can reach acceptance of diabetes and still feel regret and sadness.

When you feel you have reached the acceptance stage, you should celebrate this huge accomplishment. Then consider paying it forward by sharing what you have learned along the way. For every woman with diabetes who has found acceptance, there are many more who still are struggling.

SOUL-SEARCHING

What has diabetes taught you/revealed to you about yourself?

_____

_____

_____

_____

What positive things have occurred in your life because of your diabetes? (For example, are you more knowledgeable about food/nutrition? Have you met friends you wouldn't have met otherwise? Are you exercising more?)

_____

_____

_____

_____

What has diabetes prevented you from doing/achieving in life?

_____

_____

_____

_____

Now, think deeply about your answer to the question above. Did *diabetes* prevent you from achieving/doing these things or did your *fear* prevent you from achieving/doing them?

_____

_____

_____

_____

Do you have any regrets in life because of your diabetes? If so, how are these regrets holding you back?

_____

_____

_____

Deep down in your gut, what do you really think is the "purpose" of your diabetes?

_____

_____

COMMON COPING STYLES

As I discussed in the last section, the road to acceptance is likely to be littered with puddles. There is a lot to be learned and understood from how people choose to navigate each situation or obstacle in the road. Do they hit the puddle head on, shooting water all over the place? Do they slow down and take their time to consider their options? In this section, we'll look at your preferences for navigating the challenges (puddles) that pop up along your journey to acceptance. Understanding your preferred coping style will help you to know yourself better and also illuminate your healthy go-to coping options when diabetes or any other stressor comes along.

From a very young age, we learn what coping styles work best for us. While there is no formally agreed-upon list of coping styles among researchers in the field of psychology, the coping styles identified by Dr. Roberta DePompeii are the most comprehensive and easily translatable to people with diabetes.

The five coping styles she identified came from her discussions with families of patients with a brain injury and were grouped into the following areas: cognitive, psychological, spiritual, social support, and physical.

Cognitive copers use education and information to cope with their diabetes. If this is you, you probably read books and pamphlets, scour the Internet, attend education sessions and conferences, and you may have even contacted experts.

An unhealthy "cognitive coper" may spend hours scouring the Internet for evidence that a cure exists for diabetes. I know one woman who became particularly focused on the diet and nutrition aspect of diabetes, reading every diet book imaginable. She ultimately settled on one particular diet plan, and she stuck to it for more than 5 years, never deviating from the assigned foods or portion sizes. Granted, she lost a great deal of weight in the process, but she also sacrificed her happiness. We all need a certain amount of flexibility in our lives. When a person feels like they are being restricted from something that brings them joy, it wears them down mentally.

Psychological copers focus on internal thoughts and feelings to manage challenges. A healthy "psychological coper" might keep a journal, enjoy being an advocate, or dedicate time to talking to and helping newly diagnosed people. Many of these kinds of "copers" serve as leaders of our support groups.

An unhealthy "psychological coper" might focus on the restrictive aspects of diabetes and how the disease has destroyed her life. As a result, she might use drugs, pills, or food to cope with the psychological overload. The next section, on eating disorders, will explore this topic further.

Spiritual copers put their trust in a higher power. A healthy "spiritual coper" might feel a sense of relief that someone greater is in control of her life, including her diabetes. If this is you, you may attend worship services regularly. You may look to guidance from your spiritual leaders, and you may read devotionals and study religious texts.

An unhealthy "spiritual coper" might believe that her higher power is going to heal her, or that her diabetes is a somehow a punishment.

Support system copers actively reach out to others for support and understanding. A healthy "support system coper" might use these social networks to not feel alone and to share the burdens of the disease. If this is you, you might attend diabetes support groups, perhaps even serving as a leader. You might attend health events, regularly visit online forums and chat rooms, and actively engage at family functions.

An unhealthy "support system coper" might rely too much on others to bolster her self-esteem.

Physical copers use physical activity to help manage their diabetes. A healthy "physical coper" will actively seek out activities that will improve her health. If this is you, you might exercise regularly, have an organized home and office, and/or follow a daily routine.

An unhealthy "physical coper" might use physical violence or angry outbursts to manage her frustration, or she might fill her days with so many activities that she avoids managing her diabetes. Conversely, she might do very little physically, zoning out in front of the television for hours as a way to avoid her stress.

If you are like me, you are a combination of a few different coping styles. I know that I lean more heavily on cognitive and spiritual coping. It is good for me to acknowledge this because when the next stressor appears in my life, I can look to some of my healthy cognitive and spiritual coping mechanisms from the past to help me through the situation. It's always comforting for me to know that I am using coping mechanisms that have helped me get through difficult situations before. Just having that track record of success is comforting! Don't forget to share what you've learned about your coping style with those closest to you. It will help them to better understand you.

SOUL-SEARCHING

Which one or two coping styles do you use the most often/find to be most effective?

_____

_____

_____

What experiences as a child, teenager, and young adult influenced your use of this coping style?

_____

_____

_____

How has this coping style helped you deal with your diabetes?

_____

_____

_____

EATING DISORDERS: A COMMON BLIND SPOT

Eating disorders are increasingly common among women with diabetes. In fact, the prevalence of eating disorders among insulin-dependent women with diabetes is estimated to be two to six times higher than in the general population. We are including our discussion of these disorders under the "mental wellness" chapter because they really reflect unhealthy coping styles.

It's no surprise that women with diabetes are at an increased risk of developing eating disorders given our appearance- and weight-obsessed culture. It makes sense, really; both eating disorders and diabetes encourage individuals to pay close attention to what they eat and how much they weigh. In the world of diabetes, certain foods are sometimes viewed as "restricted" or "dangerous," and these labels take on new meaning for women with diabetes. This loss of control over what can or cannot be eaten can take a large mental toll on some women with diabetes, and the struggle to maintain control can be the first step toward an eating disorder.

Eating disorders affect women with type 1 and type 2 diabetes, women who take insulin and those who don't. While there has been less research on the type 2 population than the type 1 population, one study by Stephan Herpertz from the July 1998 *Diabetes Care* found that there was little difference in the prevalence of eating disorders among women with the two types.

There are many different types of eating disorders. With **anorexia**, a person restricts her food intake often to the point of starvation in order to stay thin. Women with anorexia often have an intense fear of gaining weight or being "fat," despite dramatic weight loss. They often refuse to maintain a healthy weight for their body size and frame.

Bulimia is characterized by a secretive cycle of binge-eating (eating large amounts of food in short periods of time) followed by purging (getting rid of the food through vomiting, laxative abuse, fluid or diet pills, or over-exercising).

Binge-eating is similar to bulimia, except without the purging. A binge-eating episode typically lasts around two hours, but some people binge on and off all day long. Binge-eaters often eat even when they're not hungry and continue eating long after they're full. They may also gorge themselves as fast as they can while barely registering what they're eating or tasting.

The key features of binge-eating disorder are:

- Frequent episodes of uncontrollable binge-eating.
- Feeling extremely distressed or upset during or after bingeing.
- Unlike bulimia, there are no regular attempts to "make up" for the binges through vomiting, fasting, or over-exercising.

People with binge-eating disorder struggle with feelings of guilt, disgust, and depression. They worry about what the compulsive eating will do to their bodies and beat themselves up for their lack of self-control. They desperately want to stop binge-eating, but feel like they can't.

Anorexia and bulimia are more common among women with type 1 diabetes, while binge-eating is more common among women with type 2 diabetes

Diabulimia, a term coined in the last decade (but not fully accepted by mental health professionals), may provide further explanation for the increased prevalence of eating disorders among insulin-dependent women. Diabulimia is characterized by a person with diabetes intentionally skipping insulin therapy to keep blood glucose levels elevated, which in turn causes dangerous weight loss. Some women will fondly recall the period just before their diabetes diagnosis when they were losing weight with no effort on their part (and little or no insulin on board) and repeat that experience.

Unfortunately, what often is overlooked is how badly they felt and how much damage the high blood sugars were doing to their bodies over prolonged periods of time. Researchers estimate that 10–20% of girls in their mid-teen years with diabetes skip or alter insulin doses to control their weight. When it comes to late-teen girls and young adult women, the percentage of those who skip or alter insulin doses increases to 30–40%. In other words, this disorder is affecting many more people than most of us realized.

Here are signs that a woman might need help for one of these disorders:

- Repeated hospital admissions for diabetic ketoacidosis (type 1 only)
- Frequent and erratic hypo- and hyperglycemia
- A1C levels over 10% (and inconsistent with logbook numbers)
- Repeated flu-like symptoms
- Irregular or absent menses
- Early onset of diabetes complications
- Unexplained weight loss
- Persistent thirst/frequent urination
- Secrecy about blood sugars, shots, or eating
- Repeated bladder and yeast infection
- Cancelled doctors' appointments

If you suspect an eating disorder in a friend with diabetes, the first step is to approach her in a non-accusatory, caring manner, and calmly explain why you are concerned about her. However, also realize that you cannot force anyone to get help. She has to want help herself. The best role you can play is that of unconditional supporter.

Sometimes women don't even realize what they are doing to themselves or that what they are doing is actually an eating disorder. In fact, I met one such woman at one of DiabetesSisters' Conferences. She had traveled thousands of miles to attend the conference and was so excited to be in the midst of other women with diabetes. At the closing session, the audience was asked, "What is the most important thing you learned from attending this conference?" She stood up and said, "I learned that I have been living with an eating disorder called diabulimia for the last 15 years, and I'm ready to get help." She was so relieved to have a name for this behavior that made her feel such shame, and to have a multitude of resources available to her.

In fact, there are many women with eating disorders who attend our conferences in search of camaraderie, support, and understanding. They are very much under-the-radar, hoping that someone will broach the topic of eating disorders so that they can listen in. Women with eating disorders exist all around us. You may know one of them or you may be one of them.

If you are currently dealing with an eating disorder, I want to reach my hand out to you. (Actually, I want to give you a big hug!) You don't have to walk this journey alone. I have met and talked with women with diabetes from all over the United States, ranging in age from 15 to 65, who are actively dealing with an eating disorder.

But it's important that you seek help. It does not take more than a few years for these disorders to wreak havoc on your body. One young woman I know who started skipping insulin at age 15 (diabulimia) had deteriorated so far by the age of 17 that she had to be resuscitated by medical personnel. She has also had numerous surgeries to correct the damage she did to her body in that short period of time. I am not telling you this to scare you; I am sharing this because many women don't realize the damage they are doing to their bodies. This topic of diabetes and eating disorders just isn't talked about very much.

The first step is to talk with someone. Acknowledging this challenge in your life—out loud—is a huge step. It doesn't matter who you talk to; this is not something you can or should deal with alone. Next, talk with a health care professional or call an eating disorders hotline. Please be aware that not all eating disorder resources are familiar with the unique characteristics and treatment for eating disorders in women with diabetes. There are treatment centers throughout the country that specialize in eating disorders in women with diabetes. Please take a look at the list of eating disorder resources at the end of this book for more information on this topic.

RUNNING OUT OF GAS: WHAT TO DO WHEN BURNOUT HITS

Diabetes is a 24-hour, 7-day-a-week disease that never goes away, and that kind of constant attention can lead to diabetes burnout. Although some people confuse burnout with depression, they are actually very different. Burnout happens when a person grows weary from the daily grind of diabetes and then simply ignores it for a period of time. Finally, they throw their hands in the air exclaiming: "I give up." I recently heard burnout described as "the complete exhausting of a person's physical and intellectual resources caused by excessive efforts to attain certain, unrealistic job-relatd goals." Diabetes is, essentially, another full-time job, and we all get sick of our jobs from time to time.

When diabetes burnout hits, we have a few suggestions:

- Get someone in your family to take over your diabetes. I have actually had my husband take over my diabetes management for a weekend. He was responsible for determining my bolus amounts for the food I consumed, dialing the dose up on my pump, and checking my blood sugar. (And yes, I gave him complete control, and sometimes he did not count the carbs correctly. But, that's just a part of everyday life for women with diabetes and I think it was great for him to see how difficult it is to walk the blood sugar tightrope all day every day.)

- Share your feelings with an in-person diabetes support group or on an online diabetes forum.

- Take a break from one or two diabetes responsibilities for a short time. Just having the ability to take a deep breath and stop juggling all of your diabetes requirements at once can provide a much needed sense of relief.

- Temporarily change your environment, if possible. A trip to the beach or the mountains gives me a new perspective on life because it takes me out of my usual daily grind. I see and appreciate things that I don't notice at home. I always notice the butterflies and the intense beauty of the skyline when I'm at the beach. I appreciate the breeze that flows through my hair and the way the sun feels on my skin. I could certainly see many of the same things at my home, but I don't. They have become mundane and monotonous in my daily life.

- By all means, share your feelings with someone you trust. Being alone in "diabetes burnout" only compounds the situation.

KEYS TO A HAPPY, HEALTHY JOURNEY

The most important message we can give you is that *YOU are the person responsible for taking care of YOU.* It is not your husband's, your child's, or your mother's responsibility. If you do not take care of you, who will?

Making your health and wellness a priority requires a major shift in your thought process and your behavior. Those who are used to reaping the gifts of your selflessness are likely the ones who will put up the biggest fight and create the most barriers when you start making your health and mental health a priority. You may have a child who is suddenly required to wash his own clothes because mom is using laundry time to exercise or attend a dinner with her friends. That child is likely to focus on the short-term inconvenience rather than the long-term benefit of his mom being happy, healthy, and living longer. When you explain the changes you are making in your life to your family in terms of the long-term benefits, it will be difficult for them to argue with the rationale.

Furthermore, think about the valuable messages this shift sends your children. You are modeling behaviors and attitudes that hopefully they will pass on to *their* children. I don't want my daughter to believe that she should put her own mental and physical health on hold to take care of everyone else in the family. I do not want to celebrate that kind of martyrdom. Let's help our children learn how to develop into happy and healthy adults by modeling healthy behaviors ourselves!

A Healthy Sense of Self-Respect

Even if a woman does take time for herself, she may do it quietly so as not to appear "selfish." Women are taught to be nurturers and applauded when selfless behavior is displayed.

Let's stop here. I want you to imagine me standing on a mountaintop with a megaphone shouting the following sentence: *If the only thing you get from reading this book is the realization that it is not selfish to make your health a priority in your life, I will be perfectly happy with that!* A colleague in the health care field used a phrase the other day that struck me. She was discussing a new concept called "healthy selfishness." It seems like an oxymoron, right? Those two words just don't go together. I guess that's why it got my attention. She was discussing how important it is for women with diabetes to give themselves permission to make their health a priority.

The word "selfishness" just doesn't feel good to me, so maybe a more accurate phrase to use is "healthy self-respect." The key to healthy self-respect with diabetes is that while your health must always have a high level of precedence for *you*, you can choose when to make your health a top priority for *others* around you.

Bringing a snack on a work trip to accommodate your insulin peaks illustrates a healthy level of self-respect. This kind of organization and planning are to be commended. On the other hand, choosing not to pack a snack and expecting everyone on the trip to stop and eat at a specific time to accommodate your diabetes needs displays unhealthy selfishness. My point is that there is incredible value in respecting yourself and your unique needs as a woman with diabetes. When you don't make your health a priority, you are more likely to be hospitalized because of consistently high or low blood glucose levels or face irreversible complications. When you do make your health a priority in your life, not only does your own level of self-respect increase, but others' level of respect for you also increases.

Another example of unhealthy selfishness can be seen when a woman uses her diabetes as a crutch or to gain an unfair advantage. For example, if a woman can't finish a work assignment on time and she uses her diabetes as an excuse, that's unhealthy selfishness. If a woman uses her diabetes as a reason to avoid difficult situations at work or uses her diabetes in an argument with her spouse to avoid taking responsibility for her wrong-doing ("It's because my blood sugar was high today"), it can be considered unhealthy selfishness. It is healthy to acknowledge that diabetes may have been a factor in your negative behavior, but to remove all responsibility from yourself or to use it as a false excuse is self-serving and constitutes unhealthy selfishness.

Hopefully, the explanation provided here will help you make a distinction between healthy and unhealthy behaviors that have become ingrained in your life. While some women err on the side of selflessness, others err on the side of selfishness. Because it is a topic that is not given much thought in our lives, take a few moments to consider your actions and behaviors.

Unhealthy Selflessness   **Healthy Self-Respect**   **Unhealthy Selfishness**

1   2   3   4   5   6   7   8   9   10

SOUL-SEARCHING

Thinking through your daily behaviors and habits, where do you sit on the spectrum shown in the graphic above?

_____

_____

_____

_____

_____

What specific behaviors contribute to your answer?

_____

_____

_____

_____

_____

What steps can you take to get closer to healthy self-respect?

_____

_____

Unleashing Your Spirituality

No book that offers a holistic view of women with diabetes would be complete without a discussion on nourishing your spirit. I often hear women with diabetes discuss how diabetes affects every part of their body, mind, and spirit. But, what exactly is "spirit"?

According to the Oxford Dictionaries, *spirit* is defined as "the non-physical part of a person which is the seat of emotions and character; the soul." Many people associate spirit with religion and rituals; others associate spirit with practices such as meditation. Regardless of the path you take, spiritual scholars tend to agree that nourishing one's spirit should result in an improved outlook, a better understanding of one's life purpose, and a more fulfilled life.

Personally, I know that spirituality has made me more centered, given me a stronger focus, and solidified my purpose. I would not have the skills or aptitude to lead a national nonprofit organization for women with diabetes, nor would I be writing this book, if I had not taken the time to nourish my spirit over the last decade. Nourishing one's spirit is difficult for women because it requires us to slow down and really listen to our inner voice. Maybe you could take this step through journaling, meditating, taking self-discovery quizzes, reading religious books, or spending time at a retreat. Think of nourishing your spirit as anything that helps you get to the "core" of who you are as a person.

The year 2007 was one of introspection and spiritual growth for me. It started with a peculiar restlessness in my soul. After hours of introspection and prayer, I uncovered that the restlessness was really a feeling that I should be using my unique skills and abilities to help others in a more significant way. Of course, that realization set me on a bigger journey to uncover what I could do that would fulfill this larger purpose. During this time, I used many different routes to get to know myself better. I spent time journaling, completed career assessment quizzes such as the strengths-Finder, read books such as *The Purpose-Driven Life,* and prayed.

Aside from this internal restlessness in my soul, my physical body was undergoing major turmoil in 2007. I was hospitalized four times, had my appendix removed, had kidney stones, lost an unhealthy amount of weight, endured a mystery illness for 6 months before it was correctly diagnosed as hyperparathyroidism, and had a parathyroid surgically removed. All of this mental and physical turmoil left me grasping for an area of life in which I could find peace. I kept going back to my spirituality. By the end of the year, I felt like I had gotten to know myself better than ever before. My spirituality involves God (though you may believe in a different higher power or not at all). I began having daily conversations with Him. One morning, on the way to my first appointment as a diabetes pharmaceutical sales representative, the feeling of restlessness that had taunted me all year long come over me very strongly. Frustrated because I had been dealing with this feeling off-and-on for so long, I pleaded with God to tell me what it was He wanted me to do because I could not deal with the spiritual discomfort anymore. "Just tell me what you want me to do and I'll do it . . . just tell me," I said. As soon as the words left my mouth, I felt the enormity of what I had said. For a moment, I felt the twinge of anxiety in my stomach, fearful that He would give me something I didn't want to do or something that was *huge.* I let the anxiety die down and my attention was diverted to the radio for a few minutes.

Then this wild idea filled my head: It was a website devoted to women with diabetes—a place where women could meet, talk, and ask questions virtually. There would be blogs (even though I didn't even really know what a blog was then) written by women with different types of diabetes and educational articles written by professionals who were also living with diabetes. Everyone would come together at least once a year for an annual retreat. There would be lots of exploring, learning, sharing, empowerment, and sisterhood. I don't want you to think that I wanted to create a "social club" for women with diabetes. I wanted it to be a respectable organization where we accomplished serious work for women with diabetes.

I pulled the car over and wrote everything down on a tablet. Just thinking about this idea and how many women it could help totally energized me and gave me a feeling of peace at the same time. Then, reality hit me. I had a husband, a 2-year-old daughter, and a full-time job. This "idea" would require a major life transformation. It would change not only my life, but my family's life as well. And I have to be honest; we lived a pretty comfortable life. My excitement waned, but the next day I found myself daydreaming about this concept again. I could picture women with diabetes coming together to support each other, laughing, learning, and having a great time at the annual event.

All of the introspection of the last year came down to *this*, and this was enormous! Uncovering my personality and career strengths, reading books to uncover my purpose, and journaling to better understand what brought me joy had finally paid off! Or had they? I kept thinking, "Who do you think you are, Brandy, that God would have such an audacious plan for *you* and *your life?* You're an ordinary woman with an ordinary family working an ordinary job in an average city. Why me?" Soon, I came to the conclusion that it wasn't really about me. This plan for an organization for women with diabetes was bigger than me, and it would serve thousands, even millions, of women with diabetes. At that point, the question became, "If not me, then who?"

In November of that year, I took out the notebook with all of my ideas and reluctantly shared it with my husband, Chris. His response was not what I was expecting. Before I had finished talking, he said, "*This* is what you need to be doing! This is what you should be doing! You have to do this!"

I had never done much on the Internet beyond checking my email, but I embarked on a journey to create a website from scratch. And amazingly, on January 31, 2008, the website was ready to launch! I guess you could say "the rest is history."

This story offers one example of how spirituality (getting to know my inner self) has helped shape my life. Regardless of your religious leanings, spirituality is something that can benefit everyone.

🎵 SOUL-SEARCHING

What does spirituality mean to you?

_____

_____

What do you think is the difference between religion and spirituality?

_____

_____

Getting to the core of your spirituality takes work. Below are a few recommendations to help you get started. Over time, you will notice how your thoughts may shift slightly based on what is going on in your life, but pay close attention to the themes that emerge in #4. As you start to pay close attention to what brings you joy, you will better understand and know yourself. This gets you closer to the core of who you are.

1. **Pause every day.** Allow yourself a mental break—a time where you stop thinking about deadlines and payments due, each and every day. This could be 10 minutes or an hour. The most important thing is that you set aside the time for this important "pause" every day. Make sure it is quiet—no television, radio, computers, other voices. Close your office door or go into the bathroom at your home.

2. **Take a few deep breaths (and close your eyes).** This is important to get your body and mind prepared for the experience and to remove any visual distractions.

3. **Observe.** With your eyes still closed, take a few moments to listen to your breathing and make note of every noise around you—birds singing, airplane flying overhead, etc.

4. **Show gratitude.** Think about the things in your life that you are thankful for and the things that bring joy to your life— friends, family, job, upcoming events, acts of kindness, etc.

5. Feel happiness. With your eyes still closed, think about what happiness feels like in every part of your body, starting with your toes and working your way up to your head. By the time you reach your head, you should be ready to open your eyes with a smile on your face. It's almost impossible not to.

SOUL-SEARCHING

What do you currently do to stay in touch with your spirituality?

_____

_____

_____

LIFE APPLICATION

What commitment(s) will you make today to help you stay in touch with your spirituality?

_____

_____

_____

Self-Confidence Is Critical

One of the most important things (if not *the* most important thing) I have learned about living with diabetes is that attitude is everything. No, I did not choose to have this disease. No, I do not want this disease. But, these are the cards I have been dealt in life, so I might as well make the very most of it. After all, I only get one chance here on Earth. I don't want to waste the opportunity I have been given.

I learned early on that not all challenges are negative. Many challenges can have positive sides to them. For example, winning the lottery sounds great, but it's also a huge challenge. Many winners of huge fortunes have been unable to handle the challenges: Where to spend it? Where to invest? What are the legal ramifications?

Similarly, running a national nonprofit organization focused on women with diabetes is an honor and definitely has its benefits, but it's also a *huge* challenge every day. There are so many moving parts, so many decisions to make, and so many women to reach and serve. I would not have been ready for this challenge if I had not persevered through the earlier challenges in my life. If I had experienced an easy life with everything handed to me, I would not have been prepared to start and lead DiabetesSisters. Just like with diabetes management, I am constantly overcoming challenges when running the organization. I'm thinking of Plan B, Plan C, and sometimes even Plan D when things don't go smoothly. Isn't it amazing how diabetes teaches us so many important lessons to make us stronger and carry us through life! Take time to appreciate the many ways in which diabetes has made you mentally stronger and increased your confidence:

Diabetes increases our confidence in our own mental strength. I know that I am more mentally focused than many of my peers because I had to overcome unique diabetes challenges. My friend often says, "I don't know how you do that. I could never push a needle like that into my stomach or prick myself so many times every day." My reply is always, "Yes, you could. If you had to do it, you'd find a way." But her words further my point about diabetes increasing our confidence in our own mental strength. My friend hasn't yet been mentally stretched in a way that requires her do something that she does not enjoy on a daily basis. All of the things we, as women with diabetes, have to do take a lot of self-discipline.

Diabetes increases our confidence in ourselves as "imperfect humans." I do *not* have perfect blood sugars. I don't even *want* perfect blood sugars any more. When I was younger, I used to strive for perfection in my blood sugar log because that was what my first endocrinologist rewarded. If there was one blood glucose recording in my logbook that was not between 80 and 120, he would begin drilling me: "What did you do here? Did you eat something you weren't supposed to? You know what caused this." Needless to say, I abso-

> "The thing that is really hard, and really amazing, is giving up on being perfect and beginning the work of becoming yourself."
>
> *Anna Quindlen, author and columnist*

lutely dreaded going to his office. I can almost guarantee that in the last week (no matter when you are reading this book), I will have had at least one (maybe more) blood sugar reading of 200 and at least one (possibly more) of 60. That's the life of a person with diabetes, and I have come to accept it because I know that no amount of anger, wishful thinking, ignoring, or praying is going to make my diabetes go away. The numbers on that machine say nothing *negative* about me as a person. In fact, if anything, it says that I am human and that managing diabetes is not an exact science. Many of the foods I eat don't come out of a package with the carbohydrate count and serving size listed on the side. Many restaurants still do not offer nutrition information on their foods. As a result, we have to do the best we can in calculating carbohydrates and determining the appropriate corresponding medication and insulin amounts. Just think about how hard it is to calculate the amount of a medication or insulin you need to perfectly match the food you are eating so that your blood glucose stays within the very tight range of 80–120 mg/dl. There's only 40 mg between 80 and 120! Bells should go off and balloons and confetti should drop from the sky every time we get the calculation right! But in all seriousness, I say all this to emphasize that diabetes is hard. No one expects perfection. And if they do, even if they have the best intentions, they are not helping.

Diabetes makes us persevere. Throughout the course of any day, you encounter many diabetes-related challenges. The fact that you have learned to "suck it up" and push through high blood glucose when necessary is a great illustration of how strong you are. Each time you push yourself through something diabetes-related (and don't allow it to stop you from doing anything you want to do), you gain a deeper appreciation for the important life lessons that diabetes teaches you.

Thinking more positively about diabetes can really pay off. A recent study showed that people with diabetes who are more emotionally upbeat have a greater chance of living longer. In the study, published in the January 2008 issue of *Health Psychology*, roughly 3,500 participants—about a fifth of whom had diabetes—supplied information about their health and emotional state at two points, 10 years apart. Results revealed a strong association between positive emotion and longevity among the people with diabetes. For every one point increase in their positive emotions, their risk of dying sooner decreased by 13%. Those who reported enjoying life showed the biggest longevity boost.

> "If you will embrace change, the winds that you thought would defeat you will actually push you to your divine destiny."
>
> *Joel Osteen, preacher, televangelist, author*

This does not mean that everyone with diabetes should just "buck up" and be happy about their diabetes. Diabetes is a disease that has its ups and downs. Every day is not an "up," but these results suggest that it is important to persevere and focus on the positive aspects of your life and your diabetes. Visualize success in your future. Do you want to be alive, healthy, and active enough to play with your grandchildren as they grow up? Thinking about your dreams and aspirations for tomorrow can keep you motivated and positive today.

Diabetes increases our confidence by making us wiser. Another way to remain positive and keep my confidence high when something not-so-good happens is to ask myself, "What lesson can I learn from this situation?" I am a firm believer that obstacles prepare us for greater things. Maybe you miscalculated and took too much insulin for the turkey and cheese panini you had for lunch. Now you know how much to take next time, or you know to eat that exact same meal and take the exact same amount of insulin if you are going to go for a run with your neighbor afterward. Everything about diabetes serves as a "teaching moment."

For someone who loves to learn, this makes diabetes less of an annoyance. I cannot even begin to tell you how much I have learned from having diabetes, including nutrition facts, physical fitness techniques, the inner workings of our organs, how medications work in our bodies, the intricate details of health insurance and life insurance, and health care legislation. Essentially, diabetes has made me a much more knowledgeable person about the world around me.

OWNING YOUR DIABETES

Over the last 7 years, I have come into contact with thousands of women with diabetes from all over the world. Some have been completely incapacitated by their diabetes, while others are flourishing and living full lives. I have given careful thought to the similarities between those on opposite ends of this spectrum.

Those on the negative end of the coping spectrum were in various stages of grief. Among those women who were flourishing with their diabetes, the common characteristic was that they seemed to "OWN" it.

What exactly does "OWNing" your diabetes mean? It means being able to look anyone in the eye and say, "I have diabetes" with pride. It means not worrying if someone's opinion of you changes after you have made this declaration. It means not apologizing for your diabetes. (You don't apologize for having brown eyes or fair skin, right?) It means taking full responsibility for your diabetes and doing your best to keep your blood glucose in the target range. (Notice that I did not say, "having perfect blood sugar levels" or a "perfect A1C level.") It means knowing that having diabetes does not make you less of a woman—it makes you a more dynamic woman!

O = Open Up
Women who are living happy lives with diabetes talk openly and proudly about their diabetes. It is not a disease that they would wish on anyone, but it is something that they do not feel guilt or

angst about. They talk about their diabetes in the same way that your coworker talks about her recent trip to Japan. She tells about the good and the bad experiences so you get the full, unadulterated picture of her trip. In the same way, women who OWN their diabetes share the full picture of life with diabetes so that those who talk with her walk away with a better understanding (and appreciation) of life with diabetes.

W = Win

Women who OWN their diabetes find a way to win in everyday life situations, especially those challenging situations related to their diabetes. Winning in this sense does not mean gaining victory over someone or something. Instead, it means creating a positive expectation or result. As motivational speaker and author Brian Tracy once explained, "Winners make a habit of manufacturing their own positive expectations in advance of the event." A great example of this is the story that Natalie shared with the audience during her keynote speech at the 2012 Weekend for Women conference. She eloquently discussed how she felt diabetes had fully prepared her to compete in the biggest competition of her life: CBS' *The Amazing Race* in 2010. "After all," she said, "I had an advantage over my competitors because diabetes taught me how to think on my feet from an early age. Diabetes also taught me to figure out many different solutions to a problem and how to react quickly in emergency situations. I went into the competition feeling like I already had one up on my competitors because of my diabetes." She went on to explain how she had already been through an elaborate amount of planning just to ensure that she could fit all of her diabetes supplies into her and her partner, Kat's, backpacks. This included making some sacrifices, like choosing between her toothbrush and her hairbrush when space became scarce.

This kind of winning perspective is common among women who OWN their diabetes. Not only did Natalie *not* see her diabetes as a disadvantage, she saw it as an advantage. Winning in life is all about perspective. Those who OWN their diabetes find a way to celebrate the areas of life they are winning in, especially those that involve their diabetes. Whenever you encounter your next diabetes challenge, think about what you can learn from it. Women who OWN their diabetes learn from the challenges in their life and use those lessons to strengthen them in other areas of their life.

N = Never a Vic*tim* (Always a Vic*tor*)

While the victim mentality was discussed earlier in this chapter, the victor mentality is what women who OWN their diabetes have. For example, while the victim may feel hurt and wounded by others' insensitive remarks, the victor will not think twice about providing the facts about diabetes to anyone who makes insensitive or uneducated remarks about diabetes, and she will walk away feeling empowered. She will not take ignorant statements personally, but instead, she understands that another's lack of knowledge has no bearing on her value as a person. The woman with diabetes who does not feel understood by her friend will do her best to explain her daily challenges, but if that friend is unable or unwilling to understand, then she does not take it personally. Essentially, she becomes a victor in every situation in life because she refuses to be a victim. She takes control of situations and refuses to allow herself to be hurt by others.

Do *you* OWN your diabetes? It's yours . . . you might as well!

"You are not your bra size, the width of your waist, or the slenderness of your calves. You are not your hair color, your skin color, nor are you a shade of lipstick. Your shoe size is of no consequence. You are not defined by the amount of attention you get from men or women. You are not the number of sit-ups you can do or the number of calories or carbs consumed in a day. You are not the number on your glucometer or your scale. You are not the hair on your legs. You are not a little red dress.

"You are no combination of these things.

"You are the content of your character. You are the ambitions that drive you. You are the goals you set. You are the things you laugh at and the words you say. You are the thoughts you think and the things you wonder. You are beautiful and desirable not for the clique you are part of, but for the spark of life within you that compels you to make your life a full and meaningful one. You are beautiful not for the shape of the vessel, but for the volume of the soul it carries."

Original author unknown; adapted by Brandy Barnes

NOTES ON MY JOURNEY

_____

_____

_____

_____

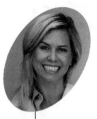

Physical Wellness

In this chapter, I will really get into detail about how diabetes affects every single part of your body. This is a really important chapter, but it can also be a scary one. Let's face it: Looking directly at a bunch of possible health problems due to diabetes can be really terrifying, and this is hard to do for most of us.

I know this from personal experience. As I mentioned earlier, I was diagnosed with diabetes at the age of 12. While it was overwhelming and scary, I really did not have the maturity or knowledge at that time to fully grasp the big picture. I maintained this semi-informed, and somewhat ignorantly blissful, state until I started medical school. My first 2 years of medical school were some of the hardest years for me as far as my diabetes goes. This was not because of the late nights and grueling study it demanded, but because I felt like I was being overwhelmed with information about diabetes and none of it was good. I felt almost paralyzed by all of this information. It seemed like no matter what I was learning about, diabetes was a risk factor for it: heart disease, kidney disease, stroke, blindness . . . the list went on and on. I just felt like

I didn't even want to explore diabetes because it was too painful. I wanted to use the ill-advised and never successful "head in the sand" technique that I had been enjoying throughout the first 10 years of my diagnosis.

I don't want this chapter to be like that for you. So let me do a little exercise with you before we continue with this chapter. I want to pretend you're reading about driving a car. I want you to imagine that you have a manual, and that each section focuses on one aspect of the car and how it affects the driving experience. Picture reading about what to do if your rear view mirrors suddenly falls off. Picture reading about what to do if you suddenly run out of gas, your brakes fail, or your headlights or seat belts stop working. You get the picture.

My point is that most of us drive every day and we are just fine. There are bad things that can happen every time we ride in a car, and of course every once in a while, problems develop. But by and large, if we maintain our cars, keep them filled with gas, and generally keep them in good working order, disasters don't happen.

I want you to remember this as you read this chapter. True, we are not cars. True, there is no manual that will guarantee we will avoid every complication. *But,* and this is a big but, there are things that we need to do on a daily basis to keep ourselves healthy. Knowing the potential pitfalls of diabetes only makes us that much more able to avoid them. I finally learned this, but it took me too many years. I let my fear of learning about the complications of diabetes keep me from really embracing the knowledge. Knowledge is power. Knowledge gives us the power to do what it takes to delay or prevent these complications from happening. If you don't know how diabetes affects your body and you don't know what the risk factors are, then you do not have the power to address them. So in this chapter, as you learn about how diabetes can affect your body, remember that learning about the complications gives you the information you need to change your life.

SOUL-SEARCHING

Do you have any barriers that keep you from learning about how diabetes can affect your body?

_____

_____

Do you have fear or anger? Do you feel overwhelmed? Try to identify any feelings that might get in the way of fully learning about diabetes.

_____

_____

_____

Do you know anyone in your family or your social group who has had diabetes complications?

_____

Does this make you feel motivated to have great self-care or does it make you feel defeated?

_____

_____

Take a moment to consider any beliefs you may have about your future with diabetes. Are your beliefs based in fear or in fact?

_____

_____

_____

_____

DIABETES FROM HEAD TO TOE

Diabetes and Your Hair

Both type 1 and type 2 diabetes can affect your hair-growth patterns. We'll get into the cardiovascular system in a bit, but in short, if your blood vessels are affected by diabetes they may deliver less oxygen to your body. This can result in symptoms like hair loss. And this can affect not only your head, you may also notice it on your arms and legs. In addition, the regrowth rate of hair can be slower in people with diabetes. This might be a result of stress, a side effect of certain prescribed medications, or even a result of one of the thyroid disorders that can accompany diabetes. Hair loss has been described among people recently diagnosed with diabetes, people who have been living with diabetes for many years, and those in between. Many sources report that hair growth improves as blood sugar control is improved. It's very important that you see your doctor if you notice hair-growth pattern changes.

KEY POINTS:
- Hair loss is a possible complication of diabetes
- It is important to see your doctor if you notice new areas of hair loss, especially on your arms and legs, as it may be related to insufficient blood flow to that area

Diabetes and Your Skin

We don't talk about skin too often when we talk about diabetes, but we should, as it can affect up to a third of people living with diabetes. Some of these problems are ones that anybody can get, but they're just more common in people with diabetes. These include bacterial infections, fungal infections, and problems with itching. Other skin problems happen only to people with diabetes and these include diabetic dermopathy, necrobiosis lipoidica diabeticorum, diabetic blisters, and eruptive xanthomatosis. It's not important that you remember these big words, or even try to say them out loud. What is important is to know what you can do to prevent these skin conditions and how to treat them if they do occur.

If you notice any part of your body that has skin that is red, hot, swollen, and tender, you may have a bacterial skin infection. If you practice good skin care, by keeping your skin moisturized and clean, you can reduce your chances for this. If you notice signs of infection, see your doctor right away to start you on antibiotics. Fungal infections are slightly different in that they usually occur in moist areas and cause red patches that are very itchy. They usually occur in warm areas where there is a skin fold, like under the breasts, between the fingers and toes, or in the armpits. If you think you have a fungal infection, go see your doctor. He or she can prescribe antifungal medication to treat this.

Diabetic dermopathy is a condition that causes light brown patches, usually occurring on the front of both legs. These don't hurt and this is a harmless condition. It is thought to be caused by changes in small blood vessels.

Necrobiosis lipoidica diabeticorum is also caused by changes in the blood vessels. It differs from diabetic dermopathy because the lesions are fewer, larger, and deeper. Sometimes these spots are itchy and can be painful. This is a rare condition, but adult women are the most likely to get it. Usually this does not need to be treated, but if one of these splits open or gets infected you will have to seek treatment.

Sometimes, if blood sugars are not under good control, people with diabetes can erupt in blisters called diabetes blisters. These usually occur on the back of the fingers, hands, feet, and sometimes on the legs or forearms. They look like burn blisters. They sometimes are large, but they are not painful. They usually heal by themselves without scars in about 3 weeks. The treatment for this is to bring your blood sugars back under control.

Eruptive xanthomatosis is a condition that causes hard, yellow bumps to appear in the skin. Like diabetic blisters, these usually disappear with good glucose control.

Digital sclerosis occurs in about a third of people with type 1 diabetes. The skin on the backs of the hands can become thick and stiff. The joints in your hands may also feel stiff. Rarely, this can also affect the knees, ankles, and elbows. The treatment for this? You guessed it. Bring your blood sugars under good control.

KEY POINTS:
- Diabetes can affect hair and skin
- Both bacterial and fungal infections can occur, and skin changes should be evaluated quickly
- Blisters, brown spots, and hard yellow bumps may appear on skin because of diabetes
- Good glucose control can improve and cure many hair and skin problems

Diabetes and Your Brain

Studies have linked both type 1 and type 2 diabetes to declines in mental function, specifically affecting tasks that require quick processing of verbal information. Sometimes when diabetes is poorly controlled, you might feel "foggy." Things seem to be worse for people who repeatedly have low blood sugars and high blood sugars. When blood glucose levels are normalized, the short-term effects on the brain can be resolved. There are possible long-term effects, however, and this can lead to impaired memory and a permanent decrease of brain function over time. It's believed that these short- and long-term effects can be slowed or stopped with blood glucose management, medication, a healthy diet, and, of course, regular exercise.

We are learning more about how diabetes affects the brain because people are living longer with diabetes than ever before, and that's good news. One study published in *Diabetes Care* in 2009 found that a 1% rise in A1C was associated with a significant decline on three different tests of mental function. So if you keep your A1C from rising, you have the potential to significantly protect your mental function.

Another way diabetes can affect your brain is by putting you at higher risk for stroke. A stroke is similar to a heart attack, but it's a heart attack of the brain. The blood supply to the brain is suddenly interrupted, usually because of a blood clot but sometimes because of a ruptured blood vessel. When this happens, oxygen cannot get to the brain cells and the brain cells can die. Diabetes is thought to increase chances of stroke by two to four times. This risk is lowered if we can bring our blood sugar levels under control. The risk of stroke is even greater if your diabetes is combined with other risk factors, including a family history of diabetes, heart disease, high blood pressure, being overweight, high cholesterol, and smoking. We can't do anything about our family histories, but we can surely alter almost all of these other risk factors. Every step you take matters, so don't feel like you have to do the whole list to make a difference. Lowering your weight, quitting smoking, exercising, and tightening up your blood glucose control will all significantly decrease your risk for stroke.

It's important to know the warning signs of a stroke because when it comes to stroke management, time is of the essence! Getting treatment right away can help prevent any permanent damage.

KEY POINTS:
- Both high and low blood sugars can affect your ability to think clearly
- Lowering your A1C by just 1% can improve your brain function

TYPICAL WARNING SIGNS OF A STROKE:

- Sudden weakness or numbness, usually on one side of the body
- Sudden confusion and difficulty understanding words
- Sudden difficulty with speaking or slurring your words
- Visual changes
- Headache

Call 911 immediately if you suspect you may be having a stroke.

- Diabetes increases your risk of a stroke up to four times the average risk. Know the warning signs of stroke and react immediately if you suspect you are having one by calling 911
- Put effort into reducing your risk of stroke by:
  - managing blood pressure
  - exercising
  - not smoking
  - managing your cholesterol levels
  - tightly controlling your glucose levels
  - maintaining a healthy weight

Diabetes and Your Eyes

We have all probably heard something about the increased risk of blindness with diabetes. This is one of the scariest potential complications. Let's talk about some of the common problems that can develop in the eyes and how to prevent and/or treat them.

Most of you know about cataracts, but you may not know that cataracts are more common and can occur earlier for those of us with diabetes. When cataracts form, the normally clear lens of the eye can get clouded. This can cause visual changes and difficulty in focusing. Cataracts can be surgically corrected.

Diabetes also increases the risk of glaucoma. Glaucoma arises when there is increased pressure inside the eye. When the pressure in the eye becomes too high, it leads to nerve dysfunction and blood vessel dysfunction, eventually causing changes in your vision. In addition to the more common open angle glaucoma and closed angle glaucoma, there is a third, more rare type called neovascular glaucoma. Treatment of glaucoma can include eye drops, laser procedures, medicine, or surgery.

Diabetes also has the ability to cause visual changes temporarily when blood sugar levels are out of goal range. High blood sugars can lead to swelling of the lens of the eye, resulting in blurred vision. Usually this will resolve once blood sugar control is improved.

Diabetic retinopathy is the most common type of eye disease related to diabetes. The retina is the back part of your eye that converts light into images that will then be transmitted by your optic nerve to the brain. When diabetic retinopathy happens, it is due to damage of the small blood vessels in the retina. If the retinopathy is not found early, or if it is not treated, it can lead to blindness. In fact, this is the leading cause of irreversible blindness in modern countries. The biggest risk factor for retinopathy is how long you have had diabetes. However, the Diabetes Control and Complications Trial showed that people with type 1 diabetes who achieved tight control of their blood glucose were up to 75% less likely to develop retinopathy. While most people with type 1 diabetes do not have any signs of retinal damage within the first 5 years of having the disease, some people with type 2 diabetes may have some early signs of retinopathy at the time of their diagnosis. It's really important to be aware of those variables we can affect that will decrease our chances of developing retinopathy, including not smoking, getting our blood pressure under control, managing our cholesterol, and having good control of our blood sugars.

If retinopathy does develop, it can be treated. Everybody with diabetes should see an eye doctor once a year. Some people may be able to go less often if they are not having problems, but talk to your doctor. When you are pregnant, this is even more important. You should see your eye doctor before you get pregnant, during the first trimester and regularly throughout the rest of your pregnancy to avoid eye problems.

Here's the good news: If you catch retinopathy early, current treatments reduce the risk of blindness by 90%. Also, good blood sugar control slows not only the onset but also the progression of retinopathy.

KEY POINTS:
- Glaucoma and cataracts occur earlier and more frequently in people with diabetes
- Everyone with diabetes should see an eye doctor annually to be evaluated for diabetic retinopathy, since early treatment can dramatically reduce risk of blindness by 90%
- Pregnancy can increase the likelihood of eye problems, so close monitoring by a doctor is important

- Tight control of blood sugars can prevent or delay eye complications

Diabetes and Your Oral Health

Last year, I had the honor of being a spokesperson for Colgate as they partnered with the American Diabetes Association during Diabetes Awareness Month. Our goal was to increase awareness about the link between diabetes and oral health. Many people don't think about the health of their teeth and gums as it relates to diabetes. But the fact is, if you have diabetes you have an increased risk for gum disease, gingivitis, and periodontitis because people with diabetes are generally more susceptible to bacterial infections. In addition, if you have serious gum disease, this may also lead to difficulty in controlling your blood sugars because infections can lead to elevated blood sugar levels.

Diabetes can also be associated with a problem called oral thrush, or a fungal infection of the mouth. This is caused by a fungus called Candida albicans and can be treated with anti-fungal medications. To prevent diabetes-related dental problems, make sure you control your blood glucose level. You should see your dentist every 6 months, brush and floss regularly, and clean your dentures daily if you wear them.

KEY POINTS:
- Diabetes can increase your risk of gum disease and oral infections
- Control your blood sugars to decrease this risk
- See your dentist twice a year, brush and floss regularly

Diabetes and Your Thyroid

Thyroid dysfunction is a big problem for women with diabetes. Low thyroid function, called hypothyroidism, is a relatively common condition with women in general. When patients have an autoimmune disease, like type 1 diabetes, they are at an increased risk of developing other autoimmune disorders. Thus, up to 30%

of women with type 1 diabetes have a thyroid disease as well. The rate of postpartum, or post-pregnancy, thyroid problems is three times higher in women with diabetes compared to women without diabetes. In fact women with type 1 diabetes should be screened 6–8 weeks after delivery for thyroid dysfunction. After delivery, 30% of women may not recover from the low thyroid activity and will require thyroid replacement.

Low thyroid function is also thought to be more common in patients with type 2 diabetes. This is important to know because it can affect your blood sugars. If you have hyperthyroidism, or elevated thyroid function, this is usually associated with more erratic blood sugars and increasing requirements for insulin. This is because when your thyroid is hyperactive, more sugar gets made in your liver, glucose is absorbed more rapidly into your gastrointestinal tract, and insulin resistance is increased. If you are experiencing unexplained worsening high blood sugars, thyroid hyperactivity should be considered. Other symptoms may include feeling warm, having rapid heart rate, weight loss, and irritability. Low thyroid levels rarely affect blood glucose levels directly, but they can worsen problems with cholesterol. In addition, low thyroid levels may be associated with fatigue, depression, and weight gain. All of these will make it harder to take good care of your blood sugars.

Diagnosing thyroid problems based just on clinical symptoms can be quite hard because symptoms may be similar to the symptoms that are produced by poor blood sugar control such as weight loss, increased appetite, and fatigue. However, with the use of blood tests that evaluate TSH (thyroid-stimulating hormone) and thyroid hormone levels and test for thyroid antibodies, a diagnosis can be made.

KEY POINTS:
- Women with diabetes (type 1 and type 2) are at increased risk for thyroid disorders
- High and low thyroid function can affect blood glucose levels

Diabetes and Your Heart

When we talk about heart disease what we are talking about is cardiovascular disease. It is often said that diabetes is a microvascular and macrovascular disease. Microvascular refers to the tiny blood vessels like the ones in the eyes and in the kidneys. Macrovascular refers to larger blood vessels, like the coronary arteries and blood vessels to the brain. We've already talked about some of the microvascular complications, such as diabetic retinopathy. We've also talked about macrovascular complications when we mentioned stroke. The complications that can arise with our cardiovascular system are macrovascular complications. When blood vessels get clogged, thickened, hardened, or narrowed, the blood is unable to deliver oxygen to the cells that need it, and this can lead to heart attacks and other problems.

Many think of heart disease as a man's disease, but heart disease is a devastating disease for women. In fact, heart disease is the leading cause of death for American women, completely unrelated to diabetes. Nearly 500,000 women die every year from cardiovascular disease, and this is almost double the number of deaths caused by all kinds of cancer combined! Unfortunately, those of us with diabetes have an even higher risk.

Recent studies suggest that women's hearts are different from men's hearts. While many of us reading this may laugh and say that we've known this for a long time, this is important news. Women having a heart attack tend to present with vague symptoms like nausea, fatigue, abdominal pain, and indigestion. Even when women do go to the emergency room with chest pain, doctors and patients often attribute this chest pain to non-cardiac causes and misinterpret their condition. The fact that women present with atypical symptoms combined with the fact that many view heart disease as a man's disease may cause a heart attack to be missed.

Also, some people with diabetes have nerve damage to the heart that can make heart attacks painless, known as a "silent" heart attack.

Now how do we use this information for power? There is an excellent online resource on the American Diabetes Association

If you think that you are having any signs of a heart attack, be sure to call 911 right away. Just like we talked about with stroke, time is of the essence. There are medications that can be administered and procedures that can be done right away to help restore blood flow to the muscles of the heart to prevent any permanent damage.

Heart Attack Symptoms in Women
1. Uncomfortable pressure, squeezing, fullness, or pain in the center of your chest. It last more than a few minutes, or goes away and comes back.
2. Pain or discomfort in one or both arms, the back, neck, jaw, or stomach.
3. Shortness of breath with or without chest discomfort.
4. Other signs such as breaking out in a cold sweat, nausea, or lightheadedness.
5. As with men, women's most common heart attack symptom is chest pain or discomfort. But women are somewhat more likely than men to experience some of the other common symptoms, particularly shortness of breath, nausea/vomiting, and back and jaw pain.

website about reducing your cardiac risk. I suggest going to the website (www.diabetes.org) and going through each of the patient education modules in detail to learn how to protect your heart. I'll also outline some of the most important things you can do to make sure that you keep your heart healthy.

First, physical activity needs to be incorporated into your daily life. Most cardiologists currently recommend about 30 minutes at least 5 days a week. Second, if you smoke, quit. This is one of the biggest ways that you can reduce your risk for having a heart attack or stroke. Third, blood pressure should also be managed, and this can be done through dietary changes, exercise, and/or medication. Fourth, cholesterol levels should be optimized, as uncontrolled cholesterol increases your risk for heart disease. Fifth, choose your foods wisely and make smart food choices. Try to cut back on saturated fat, trans fat, cholesterol, and alcoholic beverages. Try to eat more whole grains, vegetables and fruit, healthy fats, fish, and foods with omega-3 fats. Losing weight can also lower your risk of heart disease. And as we've discussed before, keeping your blood sugar levels in your goal range also helps prevent or delay heart disease.

KEY POINTS:
- Exercise at least 30 minutes 5 days a week
- Aggressively manage blood pressure and high cholesterol
- Quit smoking
- Eat a heart-healthy diet
- Keep your weight in a healthy range
- Keep your blood sugars in target range

Diabetes and Your Respiratory System

The respiratory system is another system that can be affected by diabetes. Obstructive sleep apnea is a condition in which sleep is interrupted because a person cannot take a breath, and it is often associated with diabetes. It's a bit hard to tell if sleep apnea increases the risk of developing diabetes or if having diabetes is a risk factor for sleep apnea. This research is ongoing. Either way, it is important to know that sleep apnea can worsen blood sugar control in existing diabetes. Sleep apnea can also worsen high blood pressure, cardiovascular disease, eye disease, and weight control. Sleep apnea is more common in women during and after menopause. If you feel like you're tired during the day, like you never get a good night's sleep, and you are constantly fighting against falling asleep during the day, you may have sleep apnea. Some researchers have found that after treatment for sleep apnea, insulin sensitivity improved and A1C levels decreased. Now that's motivation!

Diabetes and the Gastrointestinal Tract

Diabetes can affect the entire gastrointestinal (GI) system, from the mouth and esophagus to our bowels. Just like the nerves to our eyes and our hearts, the nerves that control the GI system can become damaged. In fact, up to 75% of people living with diabetes complain of GI abnormalities. Now, GI complaints are very common in women without diabetes also, so these problems aren't all caused by diabetes, but there are a few issues that are more common among those individuals with diabetes.

Most of these problems occur because the nerves going to our stomach, our small intestines, and our large intestines can become damaged by poorly controlled or longstanding diabetes. This can lead to abnormalities in how we absorb and digest food. Clues that something is going wrong often are nonspecific and include bloating, belly pain, and nausea.

Gastroparesis is the most well known of the GI tract disorders. Gastro = stomach and paresis = paralysis. As you can probably guess, this describes a condition where the movement of the stomach is abnormally slow. I call this "lazy stomach syndrome." The stomach empties more slowly than it should, and this leads to symptoms of feeling full very early, bloating, nausea, vomiting, and heartburn. The types of foods that make these symptoms worse are high-fiber foods or fatty foods, since those typically pass through the stomach slowly anyway. If you suspect you suffer from this problem, talk to your doctor. There are several tests that can be used to help diagnose gastroparesis. Treatments include dietary changes, medication management, and eating small meals on a frequent basis. If conservative treatments fail, there is even a "stomach pacemaker" called a gastric stimulator that can be surgically placed to help.

It's important to have an accurate diagnosis because the symptoms are nonspecific and could be due to several other conditions. Gastroparesis can lead to variable blood sugar levels among women using insulin, and treating this may help improve blood glucose levels.

Fortunately, acid reflux and stomach ulcers are not any more common in people with diabetes than in people without diabetes.

Infections of the GI tract are possible and more common among people with diabetes. Candida albicans is a yeast that can cause infections in your mouth and esophagus. It often presents after a period of high blood sugar levels. It will cause a white coating to cover your tongue and esophagus. It's also possible to get bacterial overgrowth in the intestines. If the nerves are damaged and causing things to move through very slowly, this gives bacteria a good environment to grow in. Both of these conditions can be treated with medications.

With longstanding diabetes, the intestines can either move too slowly or too quickly. While constipation can be an issue, so can diarrhea. There is a condition called "diabetic diarrhea" that can affect close to 20% of patients who have longstanding diabetes. It presents as a persistent increase in urgency and frequency of bowel movements, unexplained by other causes. Treatment is targeted at symptom management.

One last thing to be aware of is the increased incidence of celiac sprue, or celiac disease, in people living with type 1 diabetes. Like type 1 diabetes, celiac disease is caused by genetic factors combined with autoimmune abnormalities in the body. Some sources estimate that up to 1 in every 20 people with type 1 diabetes also has celiac sprue. This is an allergy to wheat gluten and often presents with diarrhea, cramping, vitamin D deficiency, and weight loss. Diagnosis can be confirmed with blood tests for specific antigens and also with a small bowel biopsy. Celiac disease can be important to treat because malabsorption of food can lead to hypoglycemic episodes. Studies have shown that these can be eliminated when dietary changes are made.

KEY POINTS:
- Up to 75% of people with diabetes may have diabetes-related stomach and intestinal issues
- Be aware of gastroparesis and how to treat it
- Neuropathy, or nerve damage, can affect how you digest and absorb food, leading to diarrhea or constipation
- Celiac sprue/gluten allergy can affect up to 1 in 20 people with type 1 diabetes

Diabetes and Your Kidneys

Kidney disease is a key topic in the diabetes world. When I was diagnosed, I had three main fears: blindness, loss of a limb, and kidney disease. It's really important to be educated and motivated here, because there is so much we can do to slow, stop, or even reverse kidney disease. Kidney disease is also called nephropathy (neph = kidney and pathy = disease). Up to 30 to 40% of people with diabetes have some form of kidney disease. Of these, about 33% currently progress to kidney failure. I say "currently" because this number used to be much higher. In fact, according to the Centers for Disease Control and Prevention, progression to end-stage kidney disease in people with diabetes decreased by 35% between 1996 and 2007. I believe this is due to better control of blood sugar levels, increased awareness of the preventive measures like blood pressure control, and newer medications like ARBs (angiotensin receptor blockers) and ACE (angiotensin-converting enzyme) inhibitors that we can take to protect our health. Hopefully, we can decrease the rates by another 35% in the next several years.

Our kidneys are bean-shaped organs with a primary function of clearing the blood of waste products. This filtration system uses millions of tiny blood vessels to filter the blood, letting small waste products pass through into the urine and retaining useful elements in the bloodstream. Having diabetes can lead to an increased workload for our kidneys, eventually damaging these tiny filtration blood vessels. When they get damaged, they start losing larger and more important products like protein. Albumin is a protein that is spilled out into urine when kidney disease starts. When protein is found in the urine, it is called albuminuria. Albuminuria is an early sign of kidney disease.

With early kidney disease, there are often no symptoms that we experience on a daily basis. This is why it is important to have annual urine tests to check for albumin in our urine. If albuminuria exists, there are several ways you and your physician can decrease your risk for progression to kidney failure. One of the biggest influences on your kidneys is your blood pressure. You want to make sure to keep your blood pressure at goal range, which is less than 140/80 for most people. If your blood pressure is higher than this, work with your doctor to get it under control. If albuminuria is present, your physician may advise that you start a medication called an ACE inhibitor or an ARB. This can prevent or slow kidney disease even if you don't have high blood pressure.

Another powerful way to decrease the risk of kidney failure is to tighten up blood sugar control. Studies suggest that tight blood sugar control can decrease the risk of developing microalbuminuria (early kidney disease) by 33%, and if you already have early disease, it can decrease progression to more severe kidney disease by 50%. So, do not get too discouraged if you do have higher than normal levels of albumin in your urine. Just get motivated and do what it takes to prevent it from worsening.

In addition to blood pressure and blood sugar control, diet, weight control, exercise, and avoiding tobacco or excessive alcohol can all help halt the progression of kidney damage. Use this knowledge as power, and take control of your diabetes to decrease your risk of severe kidney problems.

When kidney disease progresses to kidney failure, clinical symptoms may start to occur. These include retaining water, sleeping poorly, experiencing a decrease in appetite, feeling nauseated, feeling weak, and having difficulty concentrating. Kidney failure is treated by dialysis initially, and sometimes with a kidney transplant.

To make sure you decrease your risk of dialysis or of needing a kidney transplant, make sure you know everything you can do to prevent kidney failure. Lifestyle adjustments go very far. Quitting smoking and limiting alcohol consumption can really help. Also, in addition to visiting your doctor regularly, make sure you take the medications you have been prescribed. Sometimes your doctor will recommend a low-protein diet to decrease stress on the kidneys.

KEY POINTS:
- Diabetes leads to an increased risk in kidney disease and kidney failure

- Blood sugar control and blood pressure control are two of the biggest factors that influence the rate of progression to kidney failure
- Most people should have blood pressure <140/80
- ACE inhibitors and ARBs are medications that can slow progression to kidney disease for those with high blood pressure or albuminuria
- Kidney disease can be slowed, stopped, or reversed with:
  - blood sugar control
  - weight management
  - dietary modifications
  - avoidance of tobacco and excessive alcohol
  - exercise
- Have your urine tested yearly to check for albuminuria

Diabetes and Your Musculoskeletal System

Diabetes has the ability to affect our muscles, bones, joints, and ligaments. The most common place for this to occur is in our hands, but diabetes musculoskeletal changes can also be seen in the shoulders, spine, muscles, and feet. These changes are thought to be from glycosylation. Glycosylation is complicated, but you can think of it as when glucose attaches to tissues where it shouldn't be attaching. Glycosylation of cartilage and collagen can add to changes that are already happening from nerve damage and blood vessel damage. In addition to glycosylation, calcium deposits in tissues outside of joints and collagen breakdown changes are also sometimes seen in diabetes. These combined account for the majority of the musculoskeletal syndromes seen with diabetes.

Stiff hand syndrome used to occur in up to 50% of people with type 1 diabetes. This occurrence has decreased with advancements in diabetes care. Stiff hand syndrome starts with thickening of the skin and decreased mobility of the joints in the hand. Sometimes a "prayer sign" is seen, with an inability to press hands flat against each other. Flexor tenosynovitis, or trigger finger, is also seen with increased incidence in people with diabetes. This often presents as pain in one finger, along with a catching or locking sensation. Sometimes a nodule can be felt along a tendon in the finger. Treatment includes a steroid shot around the inflamed nodule or hand surgery to decompress the tendon. Carpal tunnel syndrome is also increased in people with diabetes, with up to 20% of the diabetic population affected. It's thought that the connective tissue changes from diabetes increase the odds of the tissues in the carpal tunnel compressing the nerves to the hand. Carpal tunnel can be painful, and also have numbness and weakness associated with it. Treatments include physical therapy, splinting, medications, and possibly surgery.

Frozen shoulder syndrome is also fairly prominent, affecting approximately 20% of people with diabetes. Contraction of the shoulder joint capsule leads to stiffness in the shoulder. The stiffness can get so bad that the movements of the shoulder begin to get severely restricted. Another syndrome called calcific periarthritis can present in a similar way. In this syndrome, calcium deposits in the tendons lead to pain and loss of function in a joint.

Diffuse idiopathic skeletal hyperostosis (DISH) is a syndrome that exists in people without diabetes, but occurs with a higher frequency in people with diabetes. It involves the ligaments in the cervical, thoracic, and lumbar spine. The ligaments become calcified and essentially start turning into bone. This usually is painless, and may only cause stiffness of the neck and back. Sometimes it can become painful. There is no cure for DISH, but it can be treated with pain medications, physical therapy, and rarely surgery.

Muscle changes can be seen with diabetes, usually in association with electrolyte disturbances. With high blood glucose levels, vomiting, diarrhea or diabetic ketoacidosis (DKA) dehydration, and electrolyte disturbances are threats. Electrolyte imbalances can lead to severe muscle cramping, often worse at night. In addition, blood vessel disease, nerve damage, and low blood sugar levels have the ability to lead to muscle cramping. To prevent muscle cramping, it's a good idea to do mild stretching on a daily basis and deep stretching before and after exercise. Good hydration and blood glucose control will also help. Cramping may also be a side effect of medications, particularly cholesterol-lowering drugs. Severe cramping may also be a sign of a serious condition like muscle breakdown or blood restriction to that muscle group. Contact your physician should severe cramping occur.

KEY POINTS:
- Hydration and stretching are very important to decrease your risk of musculoskeletal complications
- Stiff joints, hands, and shoulders are possible
- Treatment often consists of an orthopedic evaluation and physical therapy

Diabetes and Your Feet

When women without diabetes think "feet," they probably think about nail polish colors and massages more than infections and nerve damage. For those of us who do live with diabetes, we have a bit more to think about (although I do love pretty pink toes). The combination of nerve damage, called neuropathy, and blood vessel damage, called peripheral vascular disease, leads to a dangerous setup for infection in the feet. Even simple and common foot ailments can be disastrous if they aren't tended to quickly.

Let me share a recent personal story. My brother is really into hiking, and he bought me a nice pair of hiking boots as a gift. I went on a gorgeous hike in the Santa Monica mountains and was excited to try them out. When I took my shoes off later that day I had two giant blisters on each heel, and 48 hours later the one on my right foot looked infected. It was throbbing with pain, it was red, and it was swollen. I immediately contacted my endocrinologist, who suggested I start antibiotics right away. Fortunately for me, the antibiotics cleared the infection, but I was definitely nervous.

If nerve damage is present, it can make it harder for us to feel the warning signs that trauma is happening to our feet. With high blood sugar levels, we are actually making it easier for bacteria to grow and cause an infection. Since blood flow is critical to getting those germ-fighting cells to the area of infection, limited blood flow from damaged arteries can make it hard for us to clear the infection once it starts. The worst-case scenario is if the wound never heals. This can lead to serious infections of the bones underneath the wound (osteomyelitis) and can even lead to amputation. I don't mean to be doom and gloom, but it is important for us to realize why we need to take good care of our feet.

Besides blisters, common offenders also include corns and calluses. Constant rubbing or pressure causes calluses, sometimes from ill-fitting shoes. Calluses form more quickly in women with diabetes compared to women without diabetes. It's important to treat corns and calluses gently, because they have the potential to become infected or turn into ulcers. Use a pumice stone daily after your shower to address calluses. Never cut calluses yourself! If a callus is severe, have your physician take a look and make recommendations. If you have corns, do not use the over-the-counter treatments as they can burn your skin and also lead to infection. See a podiatrist instead.

Another common problem is dry, cracked skin on the bottom of the feet. Nerves control the moisture and oil released to the skin's surface, and damage to nerves in the feet may present as very dry skin. If the skin cracks, this is an entry point for germs to get in and cause infections. Washing feet daily with mild soap and warm water can treat dry feet. Do not soak your feet as this can actually worsen dry skin. After doing a thorough job of drying your feet, apply a moisturizing cream to the foot, avoiding the spaces in between the toes. You don't want moisture to gather there as this can also lead to infection.

Prevention is the best way to treat diabetic foot complications. We should all check our feet daily, looking for any evidence of infection like redness, swelling, tenderness. We should also make sure we don't have any cuts, blisters, or sores. Another thing we can do is make sure that we keep blood flowing to our feet. Moderate exercise helps improve blood flow. Throughout the day, try to wiggle your toes and feet. Try not to keep your legs crossed for extended periods of time. When you sit, try to put your feet up.

Another way to prevent foot complications is to wear good shoes. I hate to say it, ladies, but those cute high heels can cost you more than just cash. Ill-fitting shoes can increase blisters, calluses, and ulcers. Also, a narrow toe box (the part at the tip of the shoe) can lead to even more damage and pressure. High heels can also increase pressure at the ball of your foot, which is bad news since that can contribute to bone and joint disorders. The increase in pressure also speeds up callus formation and can lead to ulcers. High heels are often tight on the foot, and can restrict blood flow. I was told once by one of my doctors not to wear high heels. Period. It was a sad day. I was 19 and just discovering those leg-lengthening and slimming babies! However, I've been fine. I do "cheat," wearing heels for special occasions from time to time, but by and large I have stuck to the rule.

If you do want to wear high heels, follow these tips, which you really should use for shoe-shopping in general. Shop for shoes late in the day. You want your feet to be at their biggest, and this usually happens by the afternoon. Pick shoes with enough room to let your toes avoid being pinched. Break new shoes in slowly, wearing them for an hour or two each day for a couple of weeks. If you are going to an event that you want to wear high heels to, put a pair of cute flats in your bag. This way, if your feet start aching, or you are satisfied with your first-impression look, you can change into your flats and give your feet a break.

Peripheral neuropathy is another diabetic foot complication. We have discussed neuropathy (nerve damage) already in this chapter. There are different types of nerves and also of nerve damage in the body, and peripheral neuropathy refers to the type of nerve damage that happens in the periphery. The location of peripheral neuropathy, sometimes called DPN (diabetic peripheral neuropathy), is usually described as being in the "glove and stocking" regions, or the hands and feet. The type of neuropathy that people with diabetes usually get is a sensory neuropathy. Often numbness occurs, but at the same time sensitivity to pain increases. Things that are not normally painful, like the sheets on the bed, can become very painful. Sometimes the feet begin to feel like they are burning, tingling, and painful.

If you have signs and symptoms of peripheral neuropathy, you may get nerve conduction studies or an electromyogram (EMG) to evaluate how well your nerves and muscles are working. If you do have DPN, make sure you know the treatment options. Often, bringing your blood sugar levels under tighter control will help alleviate the symptoms. There are also several different types of medications that can be used for treatment. There is even a surgical device called a spinal cord stimulator that can be used to treat difficult cases.

KEY POINTS:
- Common foot problems like blisters and calluses need to be taken seriously to prevent complications from occurring
- Dry skin can be a sign of nerve damage, and should be managed to avoid cracks in the skin that can lead to infection
- Pick shoes that won't add pressure to your feet to help avoid corns, blisters, and low blood flow. Sorry, no high heels
- Peripheral vascular disease may cause a decrease in blood flow to feet, making it harder to treat infections
- Check your feet daily to look for anything suspicious for infection or injury
- Peripheral neuropathy can cause numbness, pain, burning, and tingling. The chances of this happening can be decreased by 60% with good blood sugar control
- Exercise to help prevent peripheral neuropathy
- Smoking dramatically increases the risk of blood vessels becoming damaged and causing the blood supply to the feet to decrease. Quit smoking
- Have your doctor check your feet during your visit

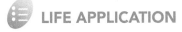

LIFE APPLICATION

Try to list five things you can do to prevent diabetes-related complications.

1. _____

2. _____

3. _____

4. _____

5. _____

SOUL-SEARCHING

How do you feel about your diabetes after reading this chapter? As Brandy has talked about in her mental wellness chapter, there are a lot of raw and strong emotions that diabetes can bring up. This is because of what it makes us go through today, and what we fear it will make us go through in the future. Being aware of any feelings that may limit your ability to take healthy and preventive steps is very important. Spend some time checking in with yourself to identify your feelings about diabetes and your physical health. Anything you feel is okay. Trust me, we all feel a wide range of emotions when we deal with diabetes.

_____

_____

_____

_____

_____

_____

NOTES ON MY JOURNEY

_____

_____

_____

_____

_____

_____

_____

_____

_____

_____

_____

_____

_____

_____

_____

_____

"The most common way people give up their power is by thinking they don't have any."

Alice Walker, author

4

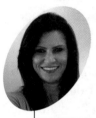

Understanding Hormones

BRANDY SAYS...

PUBERTY

When most people hear the word puberty, they think of that awkward time of pimples and oily skin. For all teenagers, puberty is a time of natural insulin resistance. However, only teens with diabetes really notice this resistance because they are required to dole out insulin doses to accommodate both food intake and unknown hormone fluctuations. For most of us who had diabetes during puberty, it served as a preview for what lay ahead.

During puberty, your body may not respond to insulin the way it used to. Your insulin doses may need to be adjusted to account for this change in insulin resistance. If you are on an insulin pump, this often means increasing your basal rate and sometimes even your bolus ratios. Similarly, when you reach other hormone-filled stages of life, such as pregnancy and menopause, your body will likely respond with variable insulin requirements. So you should view puberty as the crash course to many different life stages with hormones and diabetes. The body is producing growth and other hormones that tell the body to change, as teens turn into adults.

MENSTRUATION

Another step into womanhood is menstruation. Hopefully the early stages of puberty provided some valuable experience into fluctuating hormones and blood sugar levels. Fluctuations in hormone levels occur through the menstrual cycle and these fluctuations can affect blood sugar control. Women build up high levels of estrogen and progesterone about a week before menstruation. When these levels are high, your body may be resistant to its own insulin or injected insulin. Often, this resistance makes blood sugar levels run high, but in some cases, it causes blood sugar levels to drop. Many women find their blood sugar tends to be high 3 to 5 days before, during, or after their periods. So, the best advice I can give is to take out your record of blood glucose readings for the last 3 months and mark the dates when your last three periods began.

Did you notice any monthly patterns in your blood sugar levels? Were your blood sugar levels *high* a week before the start of each of your periods? If so, experiment with some countermeasures. Exercise more around this time and cut back on carbs, for instance. If you use insulin, ask your doctor if it's okay to slowly increase your dose a touch and back off again when your period starts. If your blood sugar tends to drop a week before your period, do the reverse: Temporarily exercise less, consume more carbs, and lower your insulin dose slightly if your doctor says it's okay.

Since everyone is different, the only way to manage blood sugars in a setting where sensitivity to insulin changes is to test and record blood sugars four or more times a day the week before, during, and after your period. You should do this for at least 2 or 3 months to find your own pattern. This allows you to adjust your insulin doses and carb intake both before and during this time to better control your blood sugar.

Premenstrual symptoms (PMS) can be worsened by poor blood sugar control. It may be helpful to chart your feelings such as tenderness, bloating, and grouchiness for a week before, during, and after your period. Charting will help you know when your PMS reaches its peak during your period so that before your PMS is most severe, you can check your blood sugar more often and take extra insulin or exercise to bring high blood sugars down.

Food cravings during PMS are triggered by an increase in progesterone and can make it more difficult to control your blood sugar. Usually the craving is for chocolate or sweet foods. Try satisfying your cravings by eating sugar-free and fat-free versions, such as chocolate pudding. Take extra insulin or increase your exercise to avoid high blood sugar levels.

It is not uncommon to feel less like exercising during your period. If this is the case for you, extra insulin may be a good choice for keeping your blood sugar from rising. Don't worry, the extra insulin needed to overcome insulin resistance during this time will not cause weight gain. Many women I know have used the charting to develop different basal rates for this time of the month. Although it is time-consuming to chart the information, knowing your own body and its patterns can be extremely helpful during menstruation. Treat yourself well during this time and keep your blood sugar controlled as well as possible.

Here's an interesting tidbit: Recent research has shown that young girls with diabetes tend to start their periods at a later age than their nondiabetic female peers.

PREGNANCY

The word pregnancy can incite both utter joy and extreme fear in the mind of a woman with diabetes. It is both exciting and frightening because many of us have heard stories about women with diabetes being unable to carry a healthy baby. It is also scary for new moms because they are not only responsible for managing their diabetes to keep themselves alive, but also another human being. That is a lot of pressure!

As a woman with diabetes who is the proud mother of a healthy, happy 9-year-old girl, I want to first and foremost say, "*Yes*, a healthy pregnancy is possible." I also want to say, "Yes, it is very doable." In other words, having your own child is not a

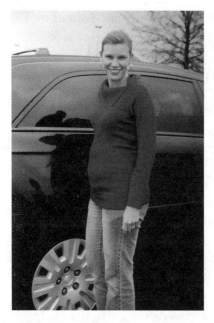

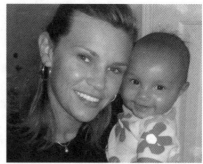

Brandy during her pregnancy in 2004 and with her daughter, Summer, in 2005.

dream that is so far-fetched it is reserved for the lucky few. There are many (millions!) of women with diabetes who have healthy children. Although some women with diabetes choose to adopt, I will focus on traditional pregnancy since that is where my knowledge lies.

First, please know that it's never too early to be working towards your pregnancy A1C goal. It's best for the health of the mother and the child for you to be in tight and streamlined control of your diabetes before you are actually pregnant. Many reproductive endocrinologists recommend achieving and maintaining your A1C goal a few months before pregnant.

The A1C is a benchmark for diabetes control that many doctors and hospitals look to as an indicator of overall diabetes control. The American Diabetes Association recommends that women who are planning a pregnancy with diabetes should shoot for the following goals:

- A1C of <7%
- Preprandial (before meals) blood glucose levels of 80–110 mg/dl
- Two-hour postprandial (after meal) plasma blood glucose levels of <155 mg/dl

Many women with diabetes who are taking insulin by injection may decide to move to an insulin pump to administer their insulin doses, as the precision of dosing and the ability to tweak basal rates is often an asset during pregnancy. For some women, the use of a continuous glucose monitor (CGM) is helpful to nail down insulin-to-carb ratios and basal rates. Some women find using a pump and/or CGM throughout their pregnancy planning and actual pregnancy helps them maintain steady A1C results.

Any changes you make to your diabetes management routine during pregnancy are part of your unique circumstances, and these decisions must be weighed carefully with your health care team to ensure you understand the benefits, drawbacks, and commitments required.

Your health care team includes your regular physician, gynecologist, your diabetes specialist/endocrinologist, and your chosen high-risk obstetrician. On your team, you should also have a certified diabetes educator (CDE), who can provide advice, answer questions, and educate you on what to expect with your diabetes during pregnancy, and a dietitian, who will be able to assist you with important nutrition choices and provide carbohydrate-counting support over the upcoming months. Careful carbohydrate counting and accurate insulin-to-carb ratios can make the entire pregnancy experience less stressful and more enjoyable, so it is definitely worth the extra effort.

The day you find out you are pregnant will be one that you will remember for the rest of your life, whether you make this discovery using a home pregnancy test or in your doctor's office. You probably will be feeling a lot of different emotions. Now is the time to buckle down and get to work; there's plenty to do in the first trimester of your pregnancy!

First Trimester

While your belly may not be bulging, your body is already changing in many ways. You may notice that your skin is a little less prone to breakouts, your hair seems thicker and shinier, and your hair and fingernails are growing at a rapid rate. Remember that pregnancy "glow" people refer to? You may be seeing it now.

Your diabetes is evolving, too. In this first trimester, as the cells that are your budding baby are growing and multiplying, your body may fall back to its prediabetes days and you may actually start producing insulin again. What causes this is a bit of a biological mystery, but it's very common. This new arrangement gives rise to a very frightening tendency toward low blood sugars, which are common during the first trimester.

Many women find using a continuous glucose monitor (CGM) valuable during these first few weeks of pregnancy, especially with the rising incidence of low blood sugars. While some insurance companies are still reluctant to cover CGMs for people with diabetes, pregnant women with diabetes are a special case. If you have difficulty sensing low blood glucose, then a CGM may be right for you. Talk with your health care team about making this technology part of your support plan.

One of the biggest emotional hurdles in managing a pregnancy with diabetes is the handling of blood sugar issues. During pregnancy, a woman is responsible for creating a safe environment for the baby to thrive in, and diabetes can throw some very heavy emotional curveballs that can elevate guilt and worry to a whole new level. Pregnancy with diabetes is about maintaining stable and healthy blood sugars as consistently as you can. For many women with diabetes, new blood sugar thresholds are set, and these new goals can seem very intimidating. Your medical team may recommend that you set a fasting blood sugar goal of between 60 and 99 mg/dl. This is the American Diabetes Association standard for women with type 1 and type 2 diabetes. The American Diabetes Association also recommends a 1-hour post-meal goal of 100–130 mg/dl. To some, these may be scary goals because of hypoglycemia unawareness, fear of nighttime lows, and a host of other diabetes concerns. Even if you've been managing your diabetes for a long time, pregnancy presents a whole new set of health negotiations.

Remember my point about the importance of having a dietitian or CDE on your health care team? Diabetes needs aside, there are certain foods that are not safe for a growing baby, including soft cheeses, deli meats, caffeine, artificial sweeteners, fish with high mercury content, and sushi. Consulting with a dietitian can help you get your head around what's safe for baby, safe for you, and easiest on your blood sugars. Even if you only meet with your dietitian a few times throughout the prepregnancy and pregnancy stages, it's very useful to review things like carbohydrate counting and how certain foods may affect your blood sugar. Armed with this knowledge, you can help manage cravings without adversely impacting blood sugar control. A little information can help you have that cheeseburger while avoiding a postprandial reading that is over 300 mg/dl.

Second Trimester

In the next 3 months, that little belly of yours is going to start gaining some serious momentum! At this stage of your pregnancy, you may feel tired, occasional dizziness, nasal congestion, heartburn, indigestion, flatulence, increased appetite, occasional headaches, constipation, nausea, and vomiting. You may also experience breast enlargement, bleeding gums, mild swelling of the ankles, varicose veins in the legs, and hemorrhoids. (Sounds like fun, right? Remember, you're building a beautiful baby, so stay strong!)

Until now, you have made very few changes, if any, to your insulin dosages. The second trimester will usher in a number of changes regarding your diabetes management. Not only will your belly (and baby) be growing, but your insulin requirements will also be growing. This is due to the increasing amounts of hormones produced by the growing placenta, which cause insulin resistance. Frequent blood sugar testing will make it easier to adjust your insulin dose and your insulin-to-carb ratio. It is not uncommon to see your insulin requirements double during your second trimester and your mealtime insulin doses increase. For those using an insulin-to-carb ratio, the ratio changes dramatically, as fewer carbs will be covered by one unit of insulin. Proper nutrition and physical activity are as important as ever during this time because gaining excess weight during pregnancy will require even greater increases to insulin doses. You may also notice an increase in your hunger levels, and you might notice some new, and perhaps bizarre, food cravings. This is very normal! Eating lots of small meals is the best way to keep hunger at bay and stabilize blood sugars. Since heartburn is not uncommon during this phase, eating more slowly may help you avoid this uncomfortable condition.

Most importantly, you should be prepared for an increase in the frequency of low blood sugars. Low blood sugars may also come on more quickly or be more difficult to detect until they are very low. It is important to store snacks and/or glucose tablets in every possible place that you may be during the next 3 months: your car, purse, desk, work bag, gym bag, and by your bed.

Diabetes and pregnancy can be overwhelming if you focus on the enormity of your responsibilities as a mother and a woman with diabetes. Keep in mind that this needless worry and stress takes away from the beauty and joy of your pregnancy. You will want to look back on this special time with your baby with fond memories. To foster a positive atmosphere, focus on the gift before you to create a healthy baby and the triumph you will feel when your healthy baby is born.

Your doctor visits during the second trimester may be both fun and anxiety-inducing. You will continue to have ultrasounds. Don't be alarmed if/when you begin having more ultrasounds than your nondiabetic friends who are pregnant. Quite simply, ultrasounds are the best way for your health care team to keep a close eye on your baby's development. Ultrasounds can be fun because they provide photos of your baby in utero. Compared with your friends without diabetes, you will have a considerable number of these photos. Today's high-resolution photos provide lots of detail about your baby. You may be able to see your baby's face or see it sucking its thumb. It is during this trimester that you have the option of finding out your baby's gender. However, don't be surprised if you notice yourself feeling anxious prior to your ultrasound appointments out of fear that a problem will be found.

The quad screen is also performed during the second trimester. The quad screen is a blood test that tests the level of four substances produced by the fetus: alpha-fetoprotein (AFP), hCG, estriol, and inhibin-A. The results of these tests are reviewed by your health care team to determine your child's risk of neural tube defects and chromosomal abnormality. This test only measures risk and is not a diagnostic tool. Keep in mind that the false-positive rate is high: In other words, many women with abnormally high readings go on to have a healthy baby.

If any increased risks are uncovered during your ultrasound or your quad screen, you will likely be scheduled for an amniocentesis. Diabetes itself is not an indicator for amniocentesis. If you are scheduled for an amniocentesis, it is normal to feel uneasy, scared, or even panicky. Rest assured that a large percentage of these high-reading cases are false-positives.

Third Trimester
The third trimester is when you will start feeling your baby move with regularity, when your pants may need to be upgraded to "super elastic waistbands," and when you literally get your waddle on. This is an incredible time for you and your baby, and it's just a matter of weeks before your family grows by leaps and . . . diapers.

It's natural for a mom-to-be to enter what the experts call "the nesting phase," though not everyone does. For some, the nesting phase is the time to clean out the garage, set up the nursery, and build the crib for your incoming bundle of joy. If you are having a baby shower, you can nest your heart out by assembling all the strange devices that babies seem to need, from the swing and playpen to the breast pump and stroller. Part of your nesting may include preparing yourself for the chaos of bringing a baby home, so it's a good time to think about pre-ordering diabetes supplies and having certain glucose stashes well in advance of baby's arrival. Order your medication refills before the baby gets here.

During the third trimester, both you and your baby will be gaining weight at a reasonably predictable, but rapid rate. Your baby has gone from the size of a large lemon at the beginning of the second trimester to the size of a large head of lettuce at the beginning of the third trimester. This is the trimester when your child will grow the most, both in terms of length and weight, and with their growth comes your resistance to insulin. For many women with diabetes, their insulin needs triple by the third trimester, so if you're taking much more than your normal dose, don't worry: this is normal. It's very important to keep close tabs on your blood sugar trends at this point, as you may be adjusting your insulin needs on a weekly basis throughout this third trimester. Be sure that you and your doctor anticipate your increased insulin needs with a new prescription for a higher quantity of insulin.

As your delivery date approaches (between weeks 36 and 40), you may see a decrease in insulin requirements. It is important to keep a close eye on your blood sugar levels during this time, to avoid any unnecessary lows.

At this point in your pregnancy, you and your team may have established a birth plan. For many women with diabetes, they're told that a cesarean section (c-section) is their only delivery option. Not true! Many women with diabetes deliver healthy, happy babies vaginally (and some even achieve a drug-free birth, aside from their insulin). If you and your partner are anticipating a vaginal birth for your child, childbirth classes may help prepare you for that experience. Learning what to expect when your water breaks, understanding how a contraction may feel, and working together with your partner on how to deal with the birth experience may put you at ease, bring you closer, and best prepare you for the arrival of your child.

New baby classes can also be very helpful. Learning how to warm a bottle, change a diaper, and give a baby a bath can help prepare you for those first few weeks. Women who decide to breast feed may choose to attend a lactation class, where their concerns about nipple confusion, latching, breast pumps, and the actual art of breastfeeding can be addressed in a compassionate and informative environment.

Other parents may have different goals and expectations, so be sure to find the birth class that works for you. Don't feel like you have to follow the status quo: Your child will be raised by you, so take the advice that works for you and store the rest in the "opinion" file.

A birth plan is literally a plan for how you'd like your child to arrive into the world. Sometimes this is an official document. Other times it is a discussion. Regardless of its level of formality, it can help a couple feel better prepared for the big day. Aside from the big decision about a natural versus c-section birth, there are many other decisions to be made before you arrive at the hospital. Talk with your partner and your physician about what your ideal plan would be. Discuss your thoughts on things such as epidurals, water birth, midwives, doulas, who will be in the delivery room, and how your diabetes will be managed before and after labor. Some hospitals have protocols for managing women with diabetes. You'll want to know about this before you arrive at the hospital. In my case, I found out ahead of time that my hospital's protocol was to put all women with diabetes on an insulin drip of regular insulin when they arrive at the hospital. I chose to not follow the protocol, keep my insulin pump attached, check my own blood sugars, and manage my own diabetes until just before I gave birth. I calibrated my meter with the hospital's meter when I arrived. Then, I checked my own blood sugar every hour upon the nurse's request, and she recorded the readings. I removed my pump just before my daughter was born and reattached it after labor was over.

It's also important to make a firm decision with your partner about who will and who will not be allowed in the delivery room when you give birth, and stick to that decision. Many hospitals have a limit on the number of people who can be in the birthing room, so consider checking with the hospital about their policies before arrival. Be flexible and open to making changes to accommodate any emergencies. Keep in mind that the most important end result is a healthy mom and a healthy baby.

Giving Birth
If you make it close to your due date without going into labor, you will likely be induced or scheduled for a c-section. Many high-risk

obstetricians prefer to deliver the babies of women with diabetes prior to their due date, while waiting until at least 39 weeks if there is no indication for earlier delivery. On the positive side, scheduling the birth of your baby can actually be a source of stress relief because you will no longer have to wonder when your baby will arrive. Furthermore, as a woman with diabetes, you also have the advantage of not going past your due date (and feeling uncomfortably huge) like many of your nondiabetic friends. However, being pregnant and having diabetes does not mean you will have to be scheduled, or be forced to have a c-section. The arrival of your child depends on you, your medical team, and the natural schedule of your baby. Be sure to talk to your doctor about your preferences and available options for the birth of your child.

If you go into labor naturally, you will follow your doctor's predetermined plan, which likely involves calling ahead to let your doctor know how far apart your contractions are. Your doctor will determine the next steps for you. If you are induced, you will arrive at the hospital at a predetermined time (most likely a weekday morning). You will be placed in a birthing room, and the doctor or medical team will break your water to start the delivery process. If you don't progress at the desired rate, you will be set up on a drip of contraction-inducing medication, such as Pitocin. Your stomach will likely be fluttering as you feel more and more excited about the birth of your new baby. You may also begin to feel some pain from the contraction. The amount of pain you feel after the Pitocin is started is dependent on a number of factors, such as how quickly and how far your cervix dilates and how high your pain threshold is. Some women choose to get an epidural early on, others wait longer, and others opt to not have an epidural (or any pain medications). This is purely a personal preference. If you choose to wait, be sure to ask your physician how long you can wait, as there is a definite cutoff time in the birthing process after which you can no longer receive an epidural.

Consider having entertainment options readily available in your hospital room (books, magazines, television, music, games, etc.). The labor could last for a long time (24 hours) or it could be over very quickly (1 hour); you just never know. As your baby's arrival grows closer and your cervix dilates, you will be asked to "push" more and more often. If/when you hear someone on the health care team announce that the baby's head has crowned, you can rest assured that you are rounding third base and will be crossing home plate soon. At this time, you will want to ensure that the person/people you wish to have with you in the birthing room are close by.

Although it differs slightly from woman to woman, your insulin requirements will drop dramatically either just before you give birth or just after. In fact, many women return to their prepregnancy insulin requirements at this time, sometimes decreasing more if they are breast-feeding.

Your birth experience will be similar to that of your peers who do not have diabetes in a lot of ways. The main difference is that your blood sugar will be monitored very closely throughout the entire birthing process with hourly finger pricks. But rest assured, it is all for a very good reason. This kind of close monitoring is required to ensure that you don't require carbohydrate intake prior to your baby's birth. It is important to adhere to this rule because food and drink are not allowed in the 6 to 8 hours prior to surgery: If you experience a complication during your vaginal birth that required a c-section (surgery), your consumption of food/drink would further complicate the delivery of your baby.

Some women have planned c-sections due to maternal/fetal issues, such as the size of the baby, retinopathy, or kidney problems. Other times, a c-section is a last-minute emergency decision to keep the mother and baby as safe as possible. Whatever the reason for a c-section, having your baby delivered surgically does not mean that you have poorly managed your diabetes or haven't "tried hard enough" during the course of your pregnancy. Sometimes, this is just how your baby needs to arrive. So don't feel guilty if you end up having a c-section. A healthy mom and a healthy baby are the goals, right?

If your c-section is scheduled, you will have the opportunity to discuss the plan well before the actual birth. Some medical teams are comfortable letting the mother and her partner manage diabetes during the birth, while others prefer to assign a doctor to this task throughout the surgery. If you wear an insulin pump, CGM, or other diabetes device, you may need to remove it or move it to a non-surgical location on your body prior to prepping for surgery, but again, this is at the discretion of you and your medical team.

A spinal block or epidural is used to numb the lower half of your body to prepare for the incision, and usually two IVs will be in place for the surgery: one for fluids and the other for the insulin drip (if your pump is removed). The insulin drip is often combined with the glucose drip, and the contents can be adjusted based on blood sugars. So if you start to drop, your medical team can increase the amount of glucose in the drip, and vice versa. The c-section surgery itself takes about an hour (usually 15 minutes to make the incision and get the baby out, then about 45 minutes to put things back together), but everyone's surgical experiences vary.

Recovery from a c-section is very different from a vaginal birth; you may have a catheter in place for several hours, and staples or stitches for several days. As mentioned earlier, it's important to vigilantly monitor your blood sugars before, during, and immediately following your c-section, as hormone fluctuations and stress may have a huge impact on your insulin needs and blood sugar levels. Some women experience "the shakes" or vomiting during and after their c-section. So have a low blood sugar plan in place, should your blood sugar drop unexpectedly. Once you are home and continuing your recovery process, be sure to follow the instructions put in place by your doctor. Don't lift anything over 10 pounds (unless it is your baby), visually monitor your incision for signs of infection, and call your doctor if you experience excessive vaginal bleeding. Remember, a c-section is a method of birthing your child, but it is also major abdominal surgery. Go easy on yourself: your body has been through a tremendous physical and emotional experience!

On your baby's birth day, you will likely feel a storm of emotions: elation, relief (after you've counted all 10 fingers and toes and heard your baby cry), exhaustion, and excitement. Because you have diabetes, your baby will likely be whisked away (at least momentarily) to check his/her blood sugar. It is very common for babies of women with diabetes to be born with low blood sugars. Don't worry: the staff is familiar with this phenomenon and adept at bringing your baby's blood sugar up to the correct level. (And because I know you're wondering—being born with low blood sugars *does not* mean that your child will have diabetes.)

Once your baby has been thoroughly checked, you will have the opportunity to spend time with him/her and the rest of your family, if you choose. (It is not uncommon for women to be truly exhausted at this time, especially if they experienced a long and/ or intense labor.) Don't push yourself too hard at this point. Your health and recovery are most important right now . . . even more important than seeing friends and family. After all, it's really the baby they're most interested in seeing, right? This is a reality you will become increasing familiar with, especially when it comes to dealing with grandparents!

Rest as much as possible while you are in the hospital, as you won't get much rest once you leave. Determine ahead of time whether or not you want your baby to sleep in your hospital room. Many mothers are so excited about their new baby and immediately jump at the opportunity to have their newborn in the room with them. Personally, I was exhausted and needed rest after birth and I found that it took a lot more energy to have the baby in the room with me. It was just easier to have the baby brought to me when it was time to feed so that I could get the rest I needed. This is a personal choice that you will need to make for yourself. I just encourage you to not feel guilty for taking care of yourself. Your baby needs you to be healthy, both mentally and physically.

Going Home From the Hospital

Going Home Day is a big day. You should be congratulated for accomplishing what many people have mistakenly thought was impossible: navigating a successful pregnancy with diabetes. You should feel very proud. You're probably exhausted, too. You may never expend as much energy on your diabetes as you did during your pregnancy and prepregnancy days.

Get ready. This new baby is going to turn your life upside down for a while, and with that, your diabetes priorities are going to shift. You may also be missing some of that intensive support you had while you were pregnant. Your doctor visits are tapering off and now your diabetes appointments may be going back to your prepregnancy schedule. For some new moms with diabetes, it might feel like you are flying solo.

But that's only partially true. You still have a lot of support, but it may be focused more on helping you parent in these early days than on diabetes issues. While you are recovering from the experience of giving birth, take advantage of all the helpful resources and support you can get. There are some challenges that may arise, post-birth, and you'll need to be aware of them (and ideally have strategies in place) to help you get through them, including:

- hormonal changes
- emotional fluctuations
- lack of sleep
- anxiety
- feelings of loneliness
- a "let down" feeling
- lack of intensive support

Before we dive into the list above, I'd like to highlight one important tip: Plan ahead. Picture this: You have been trying for an hour to get your little one to fall asleep for a long-overdue nap. You're walking back and forth, rocking and swaying, like parents do, working hard to soothe and calm her. After a while, the two of you settle into your favorite chair or spot on the couch, and finally she drifts off to sleep. You know if you move a single muscle, she will wake again.

And then you feel it. Your blood sugar is dropping. You need quick and easy access to glucose tabs and a meter. If you have to do a bunch of shuffling to get them, you might wake your baby again, which is the last thing you want to do.

Have glucose tabs, or other sources of fast-acting glucose, stashed *everywhere* through your home. If you have extra meters and strips, put them nearby, too. Your hands will be full most of the time until your baby grows a bit, and you'll want to be able to deal with a low blood sugar without disrupting him or her.

By planning ahead, you can have glucose tabs and meters available when you need them. Remember to refill your supplies once in a while too.

Hormonal Changes

Do you remember all of the crazy things that happened to you during your pregnancy? Did you have unusual cravings, or feelings that came out of nowhere? Those were hormones fluctuating (and preparing your body for carrying your child). Once your baby is here, you will go through a whole new set of hormonal changes as you transition into the next phase of parenthood. No one can tell you exactly what your body is going to do, but being aware that you are going to experience changes again will help.

Emotional Fluctuations

Emotional and psychological changes are just par for the course when there are so many hormones fluctuating in so many different directions. You may also be experiencing some pretty powerful psychological changes. The most common issue encountered after pregnancy is postpartum depression. That one alone packs a punch that can make it very difficult to stay on top of your diabetes management. One 2009 study published in the *Journal of the American Medical Association* showed that pregnant women and new moms with diabetes are nearly twice as likely as other women to suffer depression. Symptoms of postpartum depression include feelings of hopelessness, guilt, feeling overwhelmed, sleep and eating disturbances, exhaustion, low energy, and feeling easily frustrated. Dealing with this emotional upheaval may take its toll on your diabetes management, as well. Trust yourself to take those feelings seriously and to ask for help. Talk regularly with your doctor, and keep testing your blood sugar and taking your insulin, as needed.

Lack of Sleep

Many jokes are made about new parents not getting enough sleep, but it can be a serious issue. Fragmented sleep affects how you think and cope. Lack of REM sleep can cause memory lapses and make tasks requiring higher cognitive functioning more difficult. Sleep deprivation will leave you feeling scattered and foggy, as in, "Did I just take my medicine? Did I just change a diaper?" For moms, this makes a range of daily activities problematic—from paying bills to finding the patience to deal with a crying newborn. Talk with your spouse/partner and anyone else who is helping you during the first few months after your bring your new baby home. It's important to trade off middle-of-the-night feedings with others to avoid significant sleep deprivation. Even if your spouse or significant other is working, his or her presence is still felt and important for night feedings. Also, try to take brief naps when the baby is sleeping during the day. Even a 20- to 30-minute nap can help stave off sleep deprivation.

Anxiety

Postpartum anxiety is not as widely recognized as postpartum depression, but it affects a lot of women. Some researchers estimate that it actually affects more women than postpartum depression. There are currently no statistics available on how prevalent postpartum anxiety is among women with diabetes. Some worry is to be expected for new moms and serves to protect the baby. As a new mom, you many find your mind racing with worrisome thoughts: "What if she slips under water while I'm bathing her?", "What if someone breaks into the house and takes him?", "What if she suffocates in her crib?", "What if he has diabetes?" The additional oxytocin new moms have in their system heightens their response to hearing their baby cry or seeing him or her in distress. It also causes the "fight or flight" response to kick in more easily, triggering the release of stress hormones, which can make new moms feel even more anxious. For new moms who learn to dismiss these thoughts, anxiety does not become an issue. However, if you cannot get the thoughts out of your head and/or they begin to interfere with your ability to function, it's time to seek the help of a professional.

Feelings of Loneliness

As you integrate yourself back into society as the parent of a newborn, you may experience feelings of loneliness or isolation. For many months, you have had the help of health care professionals to keep you, your diabetes, and your unborn baby on track. Now, you are on your own to figure out how to be a good parent while also managing your diabetes. If you are feeling lonely, be sure to check out online communities, where you can easily connect with other moms, other people with diabetes, and other moms with diabetes. Support groups can also be beneficial. The most important thing to do is to tell someone how you're feeling. Keeping something like this to yourself only furthers feelings of isolation.

The "Let Down" Feeling

While the birth of your child is the beginning of whole new life, it can also symbolize the end of something—the end of successful pregnancy and the end of lots of extra attention focused on you. When you reach any big goal in life, it's normal for your dopamine level to spike. When it declines to its normal level, it's not uncommon to feel a sense of "letdown." Similarly, when you were pregnant, you got used to being the center of attention almost everywhere you went. This kind of attention triggered spikes in serotonin levels. Now that you are no longer the center of attention and the buildup to this momentous day is over, you may feel a sense of "letdown" due to fewer serotonin spikes. Realizing that life is full of peaks and valleys is the first step to recovery. Many people move on by finding something else to look forward to and/or finding fun activities to do in everyday life that create serotonin and dopamine spikes.

Lack of intensive support

When you are at the hospital, it is comforting to have everything at your fingertips—someone to help you feed the baby, someone to tell you if the baby is "latching on" correctly, someone to change the baby's diaper, someone to bring meals to you, and someone to help you shower. It's nice having lots of attention from family and friends and having nurses just a buzz away.

Coming home to do it all on you own can be jarring. This is normal. There is an adjustment phase. It's even common to go into panic mode, thinking, "What have I done? I have no control over my life anymore!" I have talked to numerous women who have had this exact thought at some point after they come home from the hospital. Yes, life has changed; but it just takes time to get the hang of things and find your routine.

MENOPAUSE

Menopause is challenging for most of us, but for women with diabetes it can feel like a double whammy. That's because the hormonal imbalances that trigger menopausal health issues, such as weight gain, moodiness, sleep problems, low sex drive, infections, incontinence, and hot flashes, can also raise or lower blood glucose levels. And since the symptoms of blood sugar highs and lows are similar to those of menopause, it's easy to confuse the two.

Perimenopause

Menstrual periods may be very irregular in the years leading up to the final period, sometimes with only one to three cycles occurring per year in late perimenopause. A small percentage of women stop having periods abruptly without any cycle fluctuation. Although fertility declines sharply after age 40, perimenopausal women can become pregnant, so contraception is necessary for sexually active women who do not wish to become pregnant until menopause is confirmed.

As the ovaries age, they become less responsive to the hormonal messengers on which they rely for regular function, and greater amounts of estrogen and progesterone are required for ovulation and menstruation to occur. The perimenopausal years are characterized by fluctuating, although not necessarily low, levels of these hormones. The unstable levels of estrogen and progesterone contribute to menstrual cycle irregularities and perimenopausal symptoms. They can also contribute to unstable blood glucose levels.

While the effects of estrogen and progesterone on diabetes control are not entirely understood, in general it appears that higher levels of estrogen may improve insulin sensitivity, while higher levels of progesterone may decrease insulin sensitivity. When insulin sensitivity decreases, more insulin is needed to get glucose into the cells.

The changes associated with perimenopause commonly begin about 3 to 5 years before a woman's final menstrual period, although some women notice subtle changes as early as their late 30s. In fact, two researchers I have spoken with recently shared their findings that women with diabetes tend to start menopause earlier than their nondiabetic peers, with some starting perimenopause as early as 37. Eventually, the ovaries become unresponsive and unable to ovulate (release eggs). Once the ovaries cease ovulating altogether, estrogen and progesterone levels decline, and menstrual periods stop. The end of menstrual periods signifies the onset of menopause. The decrease in estrogen and progesterone creates a hormonal imbalance that may have one or more of the following effects on your body:

- Changes in blood sugar levels
- Weight gain
- Sleep problems
- Hot flashes
- Mood swings
- Sexual issues
- Infections
- Increased risk of heart disease

Changes in Blood Sugar Levels

Feeling moody? You might assume the problem is due to low blood sugar, so you eat, attempting to raise glucose levels. In fact, your blood sugar may not be low, and the extra food could actually drive it higher, adding unnecessary calories. Estrogen and progesterone affect your cells' response to insulin. As you go through menopause, changing hormone levels can cause your blood sugar to fluctuate, making it more difficult to control. You will likely need to check your blood glucose levels more frequently during menopause so they don't get out of control and lead to complications such as nerve damage, eye disease, or cardiovascular problems. Also try keeping a daily record. If your level is too high or too low several days in a row, talk to your physician about changing or adjusting your insulin dose. If you don't take insulin, try eating fewer carbs or sugars and exercising regularly.

Weight Gain

One of the most dreaded effects of menopause, gaining weight, can change the amount of insulin or oral medications you need to regulate your blood glucose levels. You can keep weight gain at bay if you make healthy lifestyle choices such as eating nutritious foods and exercising daily. Hopefully you have already implemented these behaviors so you don't have to make drastic lifestyle changes amid the radical physical changes your body is undergoing during menopause.

Sleep Problems

Menopausal symptoms such as hot flashes or night sweats may keep you up at night or interfere with your normal sleeping patterns, which can cause changes in your blood glucose levels. If this is the case, you might want to check your blood sugar during the night to ensure it is not going too low or too high. Recent studies have shown that lack of sleep contributes to weight gain. That's because sleep deprivation decreases leptin, a hormone that helps control appetite, and increases ghrelin, a hormone that stimulates it, so you pack on pounds, according to the National Sleep Foundation. The high blood glucose levels also increase urine output, as the body tries to eliminate excess sugar. That may lead to wee-hour bathroom breaks that disrupt sleep, according to the American Diabetes Association. If you are having trouble getting enough sleep, you might try the following: avoid triggers, keep your bedroom cool, and try exercising in the late afternoon.

Hot Flashes

The cause of hot flashes related to menopause is not known. Scientists believe dropping estrogen levels disrupt the hypothalamus (an area of the brain that regulates body temperature), according to the Mayo Clinic. To decrease or prevent the occurrence of hot flashes, avoid some of the things thought to trigger or aggravate them, including stress, caffeine, alcohol, cigarette smoke, and heat. If you wake up hot and sweaty from a sound sleep, with a racing heart and a crashing headache, it's probably a hot flash. Because the hormonal imbalances of menopause make it harder to control high blood glucose levels, and a sudden drop in blood glucose can lead to more intense hot flashes, hot flashes can be worse for women with diabetes. Not good news, but there are some things you can do.

If you have extra padding, lose weight. Excess weight has been shown to increase the risk for hot flashes. You may also talk with your doctor about medications that have been shown to reduce hot flashes, such as estrogen, selective serotonin reuptake inhibitors (SSRIs), selective norepinephrine reuptake inhibitors, and gabapentin. In addition to the lifestyle changes already described, there are many simple techniques that may help to relieve minor to moderate episodes of hot flashes. These include the following:

- Avoid heat around the face area from devices such as hair dryers and curling irons
- Avoid using hot tubs, and keep baths and showers tepid or cool
- Drink cold water or water with ice
- Wear layers of clothing so you can take off some clothing, if needed

- Sleep with a light blanket or other covering and with the windows open or a small fan blowing directly on you
- Use a ceiling fan or air conditioner if you have one
- Place cold compresses on your face when you experience hot flashes or sweating
- Practice deep abdominal breathing—count to 10 while inhaling slowly, then exhale slowly while counting to 10. Repeat 10 times.
- Try to identify and avoid your own personal hot-flash triggers
- Remind yourself that your symptoms will eventually lessen or abate

Mood Swings

Hormone fluctuations, coupled with stress and menopause-related concerns about body image, sexuality, infertility, or aging can cause uncontrollable mood swings in menopausal women. Stress and mood swings can also cause changes in your blood sugar levels and make them more difficult to manage. Women with type 2 diabetes are almost twice as likely as others to have symptoms of depression, according to a 2008 study at Johns Hopkins University School of Medicine in Baltimore. That's because the daily stress of diabetes control can zap your spirits and make it harder to manage the disease, according to the American Diabetes Association. That gets worse during menopause, when low estrogen levels exacerbate mood swings, stress, and depression, according to the Mayo Clinic.

To combat random mood swings, monitor your blood sugar levels several times a day to make sure they're not too high or low. Even slight fluctuations can cause mood swings. You may also want to talk to your doctor about taking a prescription medication for depression.

Sexual Issues

Changes in estrogen and progesterone can cause vaginal dryness and a decrease in libido, side effects that are compounded by diabetes. For women going through menopause, plummeting hormones can cause vaginal dryness leading to uncomfortable or even painful sex. Women with diabetes may find it harder to get aroused and have an orgasm due to damaged nerves and blood vessels of the vagina. If you are experiencing pain or discomfort during sex, try a vaginal lubricant like Replens. If over-the-counter gels aren't enough, your doctor can prescribe a transdermal estrogen vaginal cream. According to a 2008 Columbia University study, women with diabetes who used a transdermal vaginal cream reported that sex was more comfortable.

Infections

High blood glucose can increase the risk of yeast infections and urinary tract infections before menopause. The risk is even higher during and after menopause when low estrogen levels make your body more susceptible to these bacterial infections. Women with diabetes have a higher risk of these infections because they may suffer from poor circulation. Additionally, older women have lower estrogen levels in the bladder and vagina, and that estrogen prevents infections. To prevent infections, you may want to investigate the idea of a probiotic supplement with your doctor. If you think you may have a urinary tract infection, visit your doctor so he or she can prescribe an antibiotic to kill the bacteria. If you have a yeast infection, try topical, over-the-counter vaginal remedies that contain antifungal medications.

Increased Risk of Heart Disease

Women with diabetes are four times as likely as others to have heart failure, and twice as likely to have a second heart attack, according to the National Diabetes Information Clearinghouse. Many women already have heart disease when they're diagnosed with type 2 diabetes, and those with type 1 diabetes can develop it at an early age. Menopause boosts that risk even higher. That's because high blood pressure, high cholesterol, and increased belly fat (which are linked to heart disease) are typical symptoms of menopause. This dangerous trio causes inflammation throughout the body, which leads to heart disease. Furthermore, according to a 2007 study conducted at Laval University in Quebec, excess belly fat can increase your risk of heart disease by 60%. You can counteract these effects by losing weight. In fact, losing just 10% of your body weight can have dramatic effects on your blood pressure, blood glucose, and cholesterol levels.

Although controversial, some women have opted to take estrogen for short periods, based on the 2008 multi-university study published in *Menopause* that showed that the hormone may help improve blood vessel health after menopause. According to the American Cancer Society, estrogen alone doesn't increase the risk of cancer when taken for less than 10 years. Even before menopause, women who have diabetes have a greater chance of developing cardiovascular disease, and menopause further increases the risk. You might want to talk to your doctor about supplementing your healthy diet and exercise with a cholesterol-lowering medication to decrease your risk of heart disease.

A Word About Hormone Replacement Therapy

Hormone replacement therapy (HRT) can be used to alleviate severe menopausal symptoms, especially unrelenting hot flashes, night sweats, and vaginal dryness. Unopposed estrogen therapy (ET) is appropriate only for women who have had a hysterectomy (removal of the uterus), because estrogen alone increases the risk of uterine cancer. Women who wish to use hormone therapy who have not had a hysterectomy must use a combination of estrogen and progestin together, called estrogen-progestin therapy (EPT).

Hormone therapy is the only U.S. Food and Drug Administration (FDA)-approved medicine for the treatment of hot flashes and night sweats. Many women report that other menopausal symptoms such as insomnia, mood instability, and lack of concentration are also improved when taking HRT, although scientific data have not confirmed these claims. However, the benefits of HRT must be weighed against the risks, such as those recently documented in the Women's Health Initiative, a large scientific study looking for ways to prevent a variety of conditions in postmenopausal women. According to the results of this study, there is a slightly increased risk of heart attack (seven more cases per 10,000 women per year); stroke (eight more cases per 10,000 women per year); and potentially life-threatening blood clots to the lungs (eight more cases per 10,000 women per year) for women taking EPT. In addition, dementia risk appears to double, increasing from 22 cases to 45 cases per 10,000 women per year.

For women with a hysterectomy taking ET, the risk of heart attack did not increase, but the risk of stroke did increase (13 more cases per 10,000 women per year). In women taking EPT, but not those taking ET, breast cancer increased by eight cases per 10,000 women per year. Because women with diabetes already have an increased risk of heart disease, it is especially important for women with diabetes to discuss the benefits and risks of HRT with their health care providers. Heart disease is the leading cause of death for American women.

On the plus side, HRT use was associated with five fewer hip fractures per 10,000 women per year and with six fewer cases of colorectal cancer per 10,000 women per year in the Women's Health Initiative. HRT is approved for the prevention of osteoporosis. There have been some studies suggesting that taking estrogen promotes insulin sensitivity, which may in turn lead to a lowering of blood glucose levels. (The combination of estrogen and progestin, however, does not seem to have this effect on blood glucose control.) However, this benefit alone is not considered a reason to use estrogen, since there are other, safer options for the prevention and treatment of insulin resistance (namely, weight loss and increased physical activity). Some women should not take HRT or should only take it with extreme caution. Hormone therapy is not considered an option for women who have a personal history of breast cancer, although a family history alone does not prevent most women from being candidates for the therapy. Estrogen therapy is usually not appropriate for women with a history of severe blood clotting disorders or other medical conditions that are exacerbated or complicated by supplemental estrogen, such as liver disease and certain cancers.

Did you find a lot of the information in this chapter about the impact of hormones on your diabetes surprising to you? If so, you are not alone. Few physicians or other members of the health care team are talking to their female patients about the impact of hormones on diabetes management. When I shared my concerns about this topic with one of our partners, Micromass Communications, they jumped on the opportunity to help validate this gap in the health care system. In 2010, Micromass Communications and DiabetesSisters partnered to conduct valuable research on a variety of topics, from women's biggest challenges with diabetes to thoughts on sex and intimacy. The study surveyed over 828 women with type 1 and type 2 diabetes who were representative of the broader diabetes population in terms of type, age, and ethnicity (many of them were members of DiabetesSisters), and the knowledge gaps that were uncovered among women with diabetes were alarming. Fifty-eight percent of women surveyed did not know that menstrual cycles can trigger changes in blood sugar levels; 52% did not know that menopause can trigger changes in blood sugar level; and sadly, 52% did not know that women with diabetes can have babies just as healthy as those of women without diabetes.

58%
did not know menstrual cycles can trigger changes in blood sugar level

52%
did not know menopause can trigger changes in blood sugar level

52%
did not know women with diabetes can have babies just as healthy as those of women without diabetes

KNOWLEDGE CHECK

TRUE OR FALSE?

1. _____Females with diabetes are more likely to start puberty earlier than their peers without diabetes.
2. _____Menstrual cycles can cause blood sugar fluctuations.
3. _____A woman with diabetes cannot have a baby as healthy as that of a woman without diabetes.
4. _____Birth control methods that contain hormones can cause blood sugar fluctuations in women with diabetes.
5. _____Women with diabetes are likely to enter menopause earlier than their peers without diabetes.

ANSWERS:
1. False, 2. True, 3. False, 4. True, 5. True

SOUL-SEARCHING

What was the most surprising thing you learned about the impact of hormones on your diabetes in this chapter?

_____

_____

_____

_____

_____

What is your biggest fear or concern about future hormone changes such as pregnancy or menopause?

_____

_____

_____

What impact has diabetes had on your decision to have or not have children?

_____

_____

_____

LIFE APPLICATION

How can you use the new information about the impact of hormones on your diabetes to better manage your diabetes?

_____

_____

_____

What blood sugar patterns have you noticed in regard to your menstrual cycle/menopause?

_____

_____

_____

NOTES ON MY JOURNEY

_____

_____

_____

_____

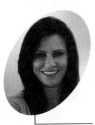

Sexual Wellness

As a young woman in college, I was not ashamed of my diabetes. My main focus was on **not** letting it stop me from doing anything I wanted to do. In fact, I pretty much talked about diabetes with anyone who asked me about it (and even some who didn't). This opened up a dialogue with my peers that I wouldn't have had otherwise. My insulin pump was usually the impetus for starting such conversations. "What's that?" someone would ask when they saw me pull out my pump during a meal. Conversation would ensue and I would explain how the insulin pump delivered life-saving insulin to me every hour, closely mimicking the function of a "normal," working pancreas.

Women would usually ask about my diet, what I could and couldn't eat. What surprised me the first few times it happened were the questions that I very frequently received when talking to men. "So, can you ever take that thing off?" Naïve to what they were *really* asking, I usually replied, "I only take it off when I take a shower." They gradually would get around to asking, "So, can you still . . . you know . . . *do it* . . . with that thing on?" The first time I heard the question, I was shocked that someone would be so bold. But I was glad to dispel some myths about women and diabetes. So I usually played off the questions with a comment like, "Well, yeah, of course I can."

Let's be clear: Sex is not just important to men. It's important to women, too. As the chief executive officer of an a organization that is exclusively focused on women with diabetes, I cannot tell you how many times I have been approached by women who are frustrated by the lack of information and resources available to them regarding sexual dysfunction. On the other hand, there are many more resources available to their male peers with diabetes. Not surprisingly, at our annual Weekend for Women conference, the education sessions on sex always have the most women in attendance. The speakers usually have to be told to wrap it up because of time, and they are usually surrounded by women wanting answers to their questions when the sessions are over. It's obvious that the time has come for more research, information, and resources for women with diabetes on this topic. The study of over 800 women with type 1 or type 2 diabetes, conducted by Micromass Communications and DiabetesSisters, which I discussed in the previous chapter, provides further evidence of this need.

A full 29% of women surveyed said that diabetes had negatively affected their desire for sex; 38% reported that their body image had been negatively affected by diabetes; and 28% said that their general happiness had been negatively affected by diabetes. It is very important that research like this continue, given how important it is to women with diabetes.

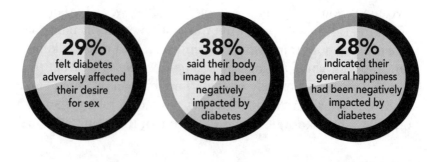

29% felt diabetes adversely affected their desire for sex

38% said their body image had been negatively impacted by diabetes

28% indicated their general happiness had been negatively impacted by diabetes

COMMON SEXUAL CONCERNS

Intimacy is a core aspect of human nature because it is what binds us to the people we love. Genuine intimacy in human relationships requires dialogue, transparency, vulnerability, and reciprocity—which is a lot of work even for the average woman. Adding diabetes to the sex and intimacy equation can sometimes wreak havoc and cause anxiety, resulting in sexual dysfunction. There are a number of unique factors that can contribute to sexual dysfunction in women with diabetes.

Emotional blocks can be problematic. Women with diabetes often have a lot on their minds. They are at a higher risk of experiencing body image disorders; some of the side effects of diabetes management, such as lumpy injection sites or body scars, can further contribute to their insecurities.

Managing diabetes during sex can create issues; avoiding high and low blood sugars or needing to take medications/injections at specific times can reduce spontaneity in your sex life. It is also not uncommon for women to share a minimal amount of information about their diabetes with their partners in an effort to avoid scaring them or turning them off. This lack of disclosure often creates more anxiety for the woman because she is hiding something very important about herself from someone she loves. Additionally, her partner is not informed on how to help her if her blood sugar drops during sex, which means she has only herself to rely on.

Furthermore, women with diabetes are often concerned that their partners view them as "less than" or "damaged" because they have diabetes. Not surprisingly, studies have shown that women with diabetes are at an increased risk for low self-esteem. Women with diabetes also often worry about contraception and pregnancy, and the life-altering effects that can occur if a child is conceived when her diabetes is not under control.

Just hearing about diabetes complications—in the media and from our doctors—can be stressful, too. Dealing with issues of mortality can really affect a woman in the bedroom. In fact, it is easy to see why relaxation is often a hard concept for a woman with diabetes to understand when she must always be "in control" of her diabetes and never take a break.

The most important contributing factor to sexual dysfunction is high blood glucose levels. High blood glucose levels can negatively affect a woman's energy level and mood, making her irritable and cranky in the short-term. When blood sugar levels go unmanaged for a long time, women are at an increased risk for urinary tract and vaginal infections. Persistent high blood glucose levels can also lead to nerve and blood vessel damage or neuropathy, which can further lead to impaired blood circulation. For women, this can lead to problems with arousal and orgasm if blood flow to the genital region is impeded.

I often hear women say, "Diabetes affects every part of my life." As such, it is inevitable that sex and intimacy will be affected. In fact, one study showed that up to 50% of people with diabetes will experience some sort of sexual dysfunction at some point.

COMMON SEXUAL DYSFUNCTION DISORDERS

There are four types of recognized sexual dysfunction disorders among sex experts. One type of disorder can and often does coexist with another. None of these types of disorders is unique to people with diabetes, but diabetes can contribute to all of them.

Decreased libido, or a persistent lack of desire for sexual activity, is called a *desire disorder*. The causes can be as diverse as serious physical problems, relationship problems, past sexual trauma, negative feelings about sexuality, or hormonal imbalances. When caused by a hormone imbalance, it is often related to a change in the production of testosterone and/or a decrease in estrogen. Testosterone is a sex hormone that is produced in small amounts by the ovaries and the adrenal glands. While the role of testosterone in women is not well understood, it is believed to have an effect on sexual desire and function. Menopause is a common cause of decreased testosterone.

Estrogen, on the other hand, is also a sex hormone and is produced in the ovaries, adrenal glands, and fat tissues. It is responsible for the growth and development of female sex characteristics and the reproductive process. Menopause can cause a decline in estrogen levels. This decline may not directly affect a woman's level of sexual desire, but other aspects of menopause, such as hot flashes, may affect how a woman feels about herself and alter her mood. While menopause is often recognized as a common time when desire disorders occur, they occur at many other times throughout the life cycle as well. Hormone imbalances can occur at any age.

Arousal disorders occur when the body is unable to become aroused or to maintain sufficient sexual excitement. In women, this usually involves an inability to maintain swelling and lubrication of the genitals. Vaginal dryness is the most common sexual side effect of diabetes in women. Vaginal dryness may be caused by:

- depression
- neuropathy, or damage to the nerves that are responsible for vaginal lubrication
- yeast infections due to poor blood sugar control
- hormonal swings

Some women find water-based lubricants helpful in dealing with vaginal dryness. Others find it necessary to use estrogen replacement. Although hormone replacement therapy may increase the risk of breast cancer and stroke, using estrogen in a vaginal cream or ring is thought to be a lower-risk treatment because it is used at a lower dose and only applied to the vagina.

Orgasm disorders are a persistent delay in or absence of orgasm following a normal sexual excitement phase. Orgasm disorders may be caused by neuropathy (nerve damage), the use of certain medication such as SSRIs, a type of antidepressant medication, or emotional issues such as depression, anxiety, or poor body image.

Pain disorders are more common in women with diabetes than in men with diabetes. The cause of a pain disorder can be physical, psychological, or both. In some cases, vaginismus, an involuntary spasm of the vaginal wall muscles, is the cause of a pain disorder. The cause of vaginismus is not well understood, but it is believed that traumatic experiences such as rape or abuse may play a role. Poor lubrication and vaginal dryness can also contribute to painful intercourse in women, and pregnancy, breast-feeding, and menopause are common causes of these problems.

The first step to getting help or relief is to meet with a qualified sexual health expert who is well equipped to diagnose and treat these issues. Since your family physician was not trained in this specific area, he or she probably will not be the best person to fully address this issue. To find a sexual health expert in your area, please visit the American Association of Sexuality Educators, Counselors, and Therapists at www.aasect.org. It is important to remember that while diabetes is a common cause of sexual issues in women with diabetes, it should never be automatically assumed to be the culprit. Tests should be performed to rule out non-diabetes–related issues as well. Treatment will depend upon whether the cause of your dysfunction is emotional or physical.

CONTRACEPTION

Women with diabetes should be extra cautious about unplanned pregnancies because of the implications of poor blood glucose control on an unborn child. There are a number of contraceptive choices available to women with diabetes, each with their own advantages and disadvantages.

Hormonal methods of birth control prevent pregnancy by preventing ovulation. Hormonal methods are available as pills, patches, vaginal rings, and injections. Hormonal contraceptives are about 95–99% effective.

There are two types of birth control pills on the market today: pills that contain estrogen and progesterone and pills that contain only progesterone (called mini pills). A newer form of oral contraceptive is based on a 90-day cycle rather than 28 days. This means you only have four periods a year. Hormones can also be given in a patch, through a small circular device (ring) inserted into your vagina, or by injection.

The patch contains both estrogen and progesterone. You leave it on for 21 days and then remove it for 7 days. The vaginal ring also contains estrogen and progesterone. You insert it

RECOMMENDATIONS FOR HORMONAL CONTRACEPTIVE USE

1. Hormonal contraceptives may affect your insulin sensitivity at certain times of the month. The steady dose of hormones may or may not keep blood glucose swings to a minimum.

2. Check your blood glucose levels frequently, especially during the first couple of months, to identify blood sugar swings caused by the contraceptive. Some women need to slightly increase their insulin dose. By keeping complete records, you and your health care team can decide whether you need to make changes in food, activity, or diabetes medication.

3. Have your A1C, blood pressure, cholesterol, and triglyceride levels checked 3 months after you go on the pill to ensure that they are not adversely affected by pill use.

4. If you are over 35 and smoke, or if you have a history of heart disease, stroke, high blood pressure, peripheral vessel disease, or blood clots, hormonal contraceptives may be too risky for you.

5. Hormonal contraceptives don't work well for everyone. For some, the blood sugar swings are too much to manage. If this happens to you, rest assured that it is not your fault and you are not a failure. There are other contraceptive options for you.

deep into your vagina and leave it there for 21 days. The injection is called Depo-Provera and contains only progesterone. It is given at your provider's office every 3 months. Before committing to any long-lasting method, you may want to try a progesterone-only pill, which you can stop at any time, to see how you respond.

As a woman with diabetes, it is especially important to be aware of the impact any kind of hormonal imbalance can have on your body's overall function. Women with diabetes face more issues when altering their hormone system because the hormone system can have a dramatic impact on a woman's endocrine system.

An IUD is a small T-shaped object that is placed into the uterus by a doctor. IUDs prevent sperm from reaching the egg or from implanting in the uterus. One type contains copper and others contain progesterone. IUDs can remain in place for 1, 5, or 10 years, depending on the type. IUDs are generally recommended for women who have had one or more children. When properly inserted and retained, IUDs are about 95–98% effective in preventing pregnancy. It's important to know whether the IUD you choose includes hormones. If it does, test your blood sugar frequently during the first 3 months to assess the IUD's impact on your insulin sensitivity and blood glucose levels.

Barrier methods of birth control include the diaphragm, sponge, cervical cap, and condoms. Barrier methods prevent the sperm from reaching the egg. The diaphragm is a shallow rubber cup that fits tightly over the cervix, the entrance to the uterus. The diaphragm is coated with spermicidal jelly before you insert it. The diaphragm is put into place just before intercourse and needs to be kept in place for at least 6 hours after intercourse and then removed. It is 80 to 94% effective in preventing pregnancy. The effectiveness depends on the user's ability to place the device correctly, use the spermicidal jelly, and leave it in place for the allotted time. Your gynecologist will fit your diaphragm, teach you how to place it properly, and check to be sure it is covering the cervix.

The sponge contains spermicidal jelly and is placed into the vagina over the cervix. It can be inserted up to 24 hours before intercourse and needs to be left in place for 6 hours afterward. Sponges are 80–91% effective.

The cervical cap is a small, thimble-shaped barrier device that fits tightly over the cervix to prevent sperm from entering the uterus. It is used with spermicidal jelly.

The female condom is another barrier method of contraception. It is a larger type of condom that you insert into your vagina up to 8 hours before intercourse. You remove it afterward, taking the sperm with it. It can also help protect against sexually transmitted diseases. It is 74–79% effective.

Spermicides work by killing sperm and can be purchased without a prescription. There are several types: foam, gel, cream, suppository, or tablet. They can be used alone or to increase the effectiveness of barrier methods. They are 72–90% effective.

With *nonsurgical sterilization*, a doctor places soft, flexible inserts through the body's natural pathways (vagina, cervix, and uterus) and into your fallopian tubes. (Essure is currently the only nonsurgical sterilization option available.) The very tip of the device remains outside the fallopian tube, which provides you and your doctor with immediate visual confirmation of placement. During the 3 months after the procedure, your body and the inserts work together to form a natural barrier that prevents sperm from reaching the egg. During this period, you must continue using another form of birth control (other than an IUD). After 3 months, it's time to get an Essure Confirmation Test to verify you're protected from the worries of unplanned pregnancy. The test uses a dye and special type of X-ray to ensure that both the inserts are in place and the fallopian tubes are completely blocked. Unlike birth control pills, patches, rings, and some forms of IUDs, Essure does not contain hormones to interfere with your natural menstrual cycle, so your periods should more or less continue in their natural state.

Surgical sterilization also offers a number of options for both men and women who do not intend to have children in the future. For the male partner, vasectomy is an option if he is certain he no longer wants to have children. A vasectomy ensures that no sperm is released from the man's penis when he ejaculates. Usually performed by a surgeon or urologist under local anesthesia, the procedure is usually completed in less than 15 minutes. After trying multiple birth control pills and an IUD, I came to realize that the hormones in all of these affected my blood sugar levels too much. My husband, Chris, and I opted for him to have a vasectomy. Although many men do not readily jump on this option, it was a great choice for us, since we decided we were not going to try for any more children. Vasectomies can be reversed, although it is costly. In women, surgical sterilization is often referred to as having her "tubes tied" or a "tubal." A tubal ligation blocks a woman's fallopian tubes. As a result of the procedure, about 1 inch of each tube is blocked off. An egg can no longer travel down the tube to the uterus, and sperm cannot make contact with the egg. Tubal ligation should have no effect on a woman's menstrual cycle or hormone production. It can be performed under local, regional, or general anesthesia as outpatient surgery and is usually completed in 10 to 45 minutes.

Has your physician ever talked with you about how diabetes can affect your sex life? Chances are, the answer is no. Sexual issues for women with diabetes have been kept in the dark for decades. Here's a suggestion for starting that dialogue: "Doctor, I have something personal that I'd like to discuss with you today. I was wondering, can my diabetes affect my experience in the bedroom? I'm having some challenges enjoying intimacy, and I wonder if diabetes has something to do with this."

The good news is that women who accept their diabetes diagnosis appear less likely to develop sexual disorders. So, an important step in avoiding sexual dysfunction is getting to acceptance. Of course, that is much easier said than done. Other things you can do to reduce your chance for sexual dysfunction include getting your blood sugar under control, lowering high blood pressure, lowering high cholesterol, lowering high triglyceride levels, staying physically active, and eating a healthy diet.

TIPS FOR BETTER SEX

- Use a water-based vaginal lubricant (bought over-the-counter at the pharmacy)

- Do Kegel exercises every day (Kegel exercises are best described as contracting and relaxing the muscles that control urine flow)

- Use yoga/meditation classes to reduce stress

- Get screened for depression

- Lose weight. A recent Duke University study revealed that shedding weight (17.5% of body weight) helped obese men and women feel better about sex

- Take some time to educate your partner on what to look for (low blood sugar during sex) and how you would like him/her to help you if/when a low occurs

- Explain the importance of testing your blood sugar before and after sex and make him/her part of the process

- Talk openly with your partner about any issues or discomfort you are feeling before/during/after sex and problem-solve about ways to solve the issue. If the things you try don't work, explain the importance of getting to the bottom of the issue by meeting with a sexual health expert

CONSIDER USING THE FOLLOWING SCRIPT WITH YOUR PARTNER:

"I want you to know that our relationship is very important to me. I appreciate your willingness to problem-solve with me to address concerns as they arise. As you know, sex is not an easy topic for me to talk about, but I know it's important to the health of our relationship. Recently, I have been experiencing _____ in the bedroom and I'd like for us to talk about some potential solutions. This is not about placing blame on either one of us, but about keeping our lines of communication open so that we both enjoy our quality time together."

TEN THINGS POTENTIAL PARTNERS WONDER WHEN IT COMES TO SEX WITH WOMEN WHO HAVE DIABETES

10. Does sharing sex with you increase my odds of having diabetes in any way?

9. Can you have sex with an insulin pump on?

8. Why do you have to check your blood sugar so many times during the day?

7. Can you have children?

6. Is it harder for you to get pregnant?

5. Will you have sexual problems like the men with diabetes in all of those Viagra commercials?

4. How likely is it that you will have a low blood sugar during intimacy, and what do I do?

3. Why do you act so annoyed every time I ask you what your blood sugar is?

2. How will I know if your bad mood is related to a high or low blood sugar or something else entirely?

1. How do you want me to be involved in your day-to-day diabetes management?

TEN THINGS WOMEN WITH DIABETES WANT THEIR SEX PARTNERS TO KNOW ABOUT THEM

10. You *cannot* get diabetes from having sex with me. It is not contagious.

9. During sex, I have the choice of either removing my insulin pump for a 30-minute interval or leaving it on during sex.

8. Diabetes *will not* stop me from having children. If I choose to have children, I can! Women with diabetes do not have more difficulty getting pregnant, but having my blood sugar under control helps the process (and the health of my unborn child).

7. Diabetes is only one part of me. There is so much more to me than my diabetes, so please don't look at me as a "diabetic." Instead, look at me as a woman, wife, sister, mother who just happens to have diabetes.

6. Sex is a form of physical activity and any form of physical activity has the potential to lower my blood sugar level to dangerous levels. So, if I start acting weird or nonresponsive during sex, quickly get me something sweet to eat or drink (or give me glucose tablets).

5. Contrary to popular belief, people with diabetes do not have different nutrition recommendations from everyone else. (We *do* need to be aware of the amount of carbohydrate we are consuming, but it's not in anyone's best interest to eat a diet full of carbohydrates, right?) In fact, just as you are supposed to eat healthy foods, so am I.

4. Open up lines of communication by asking me how you can better support me in my diabetes management. Carrying a lifelong responsibility like diabetes all alone can become overwhelming, so it's good to have another's support from time to time.

3. Please do not ask me the following questions: "What is your blood sugar level?" or "Should you be eating that?" Unless I am in an emergency situation, asking about my blood sugar level is equivalent to asking me how much I weigh today. (Refer back to #4.)

2. As women, we don't want diabetes to take anything away from us or stop us from doing anything. We also don't want to be "pitied" by anyone because we have diabetes.

1. Understand that, on occasion, my mood may be related to my blood sugar level, but please, do not always relate my mood to my diabetes.

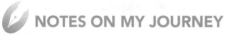 **NOTES ON MY JOURNEY**

_____

_____

_____

_____

_____

_____

_____

_____

_____

_____

_____

_____

_____

6

Creating Better Relationships

BRANDY SAYS...

I recall hearing one of my DiabetesSisters say, "Diabetes affects . . . everything. It's not just your health. It affects your relationships, your emotions, other parts of your body. It just affects everything!" Over time, I have seen more clearly what she meant. Of course, I'd like to think that diabetes doesn't affect my relationships, but I would be fooling myself to really believe it. In an effort to be strong, independent women, we often minimize the impact diabetes has on our lives. This is part of our survival. No one wants to be weak or "less than" because of diabetes. No woman wants to think about diabetes stopping her from being Supermom or Superwife. After all, we all say that diabetes shouldn't stop us from doing anything, right? So, in an effort to *be all* and *do all,* we often put diabetes on the back burner or underestimate its impact on our lives.

The reality is that diabetes doesn't just affect the person with diabetes. Diabetes affects our loved ones, often more than we even realize. They spend a great deal of time worrying about us. Have you ever thought about what goes through the minds of your loved ones regarding your diabetes?

My husband, Chris, is the strong, silent type, so before starting DiabetesSisters we had not had many deep conversations about his feelings regarding my diabetes. Recently, I asked him to write down his thoughts in a letter. As you'll see, it was quite revealing.

Dear Diabetes,

We met back in 1996 and I really did not know much about you at the time. When Brandy told me about you, I thought, "Surely not." The only people I knew who had diabetes at that time were old and overweight. Although I hate admitting it now, the thought did cross my mind that Brandy may not be able to have children and her feet would likely have to be amputated at some point in her life. The stereotypes were alive in me.

In the African-American culture, diabetes is referred to as "the sugar," so I thought that the best way to care for someone who had diabetes was to keep all sugar away from her. I was very wrong about that. Although I had lots of negative and incorrect ideas about you, I felt too strongly about Brandy to let you stop me from getting to know her. It's ironic, considering how much of a tug-of-war we would be in during later years over "control" in Brandy's life.

For the first 5 years I knew you, Brandy watched over you and I rarely interacted with you. She talked about you after doctor visits sometimes or when you caused her to have a low blood sugar or when she met someone else who had you. I felt indifferent toward you back then. But I know the exact date when you upset me for the first time. It was October 5, 2001—the day I proposed to Brandy. I spent a lot of time planning out the perfect proposal, and you stepped in at the last minute and ruined it.

As I got down on one knee and asked her the important question, "Will you marry me?" I was met with every man's wedding proposal nightmare . . . a long pause, a puzzled look, and no response. I didn't know what was going on. My heart was pounding, so I asked again. This time, I was met with the shaky words, "Yes, but I'm low." I rushed to the kitchen and came back with juice, but your damage was already done. You managed to mess up one of the most memorable moments of Brandy's life. Twelve years later, I still hold some resentment about it.

A few years later, in 2004, Brandy's pregnancy brought you out in full force. I heard about you on almost a daily basis and we couldn't attend a doctor's visit without talking about you. On the downside, because of you, Brandy's pregnancy was considered "high-risk" and everything was monitored very closely. If any number was slightly off, the doctors went into disaster mode. I saw how this put extra stress on Brandy mentally and physically.

In my mind, you were a pretty big burden for Brandy to carry during pregnancy, though I know she would not agree with me. In the years following our daughter's birth, Brandy endured a number of random illnesses like hyperparathyroidism (including surgery to remove a parathyroid), appendicitis, kidney stones, thyroid goiters (and surgery to remove her thyroid), thyroid cancer, and hypothyroidism.

Watching Brandy endure all of this over the years is what led me to the conclusion a few years ago that I did not want to try to have any

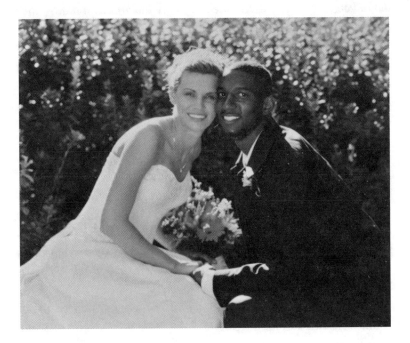

more children. We were blessed to have a beautiful, healthy daughter and I did not want to put Brandy's body through any more than it had already been through. Having her around to grow old with is a lot more important to me than having another child.

I have known you for 18 years now and our relationship has had its ups and downs. Ignorance was bliss in the beginning. Now, I worry when Brandy goes on business trips or when she exercises alone. What worries me the most is her having a low blood sugar while driving. I doubt Brandy knows how much I think about these scenarios. As her husband, it is my job to protect Brandy from harm. But you, diabetes, make protecting my family difficult at times. You take away my control in protecting her and you often remind me that you are in control—like when we have plans for a date night and you sabotage it with a high reading.

It upsets me when you take away Brandy's mental function, even for brief periods, like during low blood sugars. She is an intelligent, capable woman and I know how much it embarrasses her. My biggest fear is that you will take Brandy from me with a low blood sugar one day. Then, I will have to live the rest of my life knowing that I failed miserably in protecting her.

Life with you hasn't been all negative. Through you, Brandy has been able to find her purpose. You inspired her to take better care of herself both physically and mentally, and you compelled her to share her knowledge and experience with diabetes with other women. Without you, diabetes, there would be no DiabetesSisters.

You have also inspired me. I have learned more and talked more about diabetes in the last 5 years than I did the entire first decade I knew you. Not long ago, I took over managing you for an entire weekend. Until then, I only understood one-tenth of how stressful you are. That weekend, I learned that managing you is equivalent to caring for another child or having another job. All of these experiences pushed me to do more to help Brandy and others who are dealing with diabetes, so I started a program a few years ago to help the partners/spouses of the DiabetesSisters' members.

I want you to know that you definitely have not stopped me or Brandy. In fact, you propelled both of us to do positive activities that help others deal with you. You could have been an obstacle, but we didn't let that happen. Now I can thank you for all that we have learned from you.

In health and wellness,
Chris Barnes

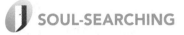 SOUL-SEARCHING

If you asked them right now, how do you think your closest loved ones would say your diabetes has affected him/her?

_____

_____

_____

_____

LIFE APPLICATION

Over the next week, spend some time talking with your loved ones. Use the following questions to uncover their innermost feelings.

- What concerns you the most about my diabetes?
- When do you find yourself worrying about my diabetes?
- What are you most proud of regarding my diabetes?
- What is your greatest fear about my diabetes?
- How would you feel if you were told today that you had diabetes?
- What do you wish you had known about diabetes when I was first diagnosed?

FRIENDSHIPS

Friendships are a big part of our teenage years. Friends remain important, and even essential, for a happy, healthy life beyond

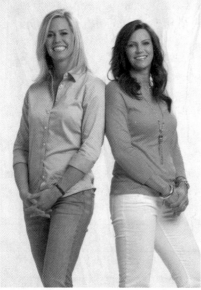

Kelly Campbell

the teen years. By examining one's teenage years, you can see how relationship patterns evolve early on among people with diabetes.

For example, one study that followed 14-year-old teenagers with and without diabetes for 4 years found that healthy adolescents were more likely to develop romantic relationships and to do so sooner than adolescents with diabetes. A 2007 study published in *Society for Adolescent Medicine* found that, for adolescents with diabetes, negative relations with friends were inversely related to psychological health and also predicted a decline in psychological health over time. These negative relationships also played a role in poor metabolic control and a deterioration of such control over time.

To those who lived with diabetes through the turbulent teenage years, these research findings are probably not surprising. Friends are important whether you have diabetes or not, yet maintaining friendships may be more difficult when you have diabetes. With so many things competing for our time and attention, diabetes management sometimes replaces one or more of the "friend" slots in life. Although we can talk with "healthy" women about other topics—fashion, children, careers, vacations—there is always an important aspect of our lives that our friends without diabetes just won't understand. That's why it is important to find other people, and especially women, with diabetes to share and learn from. Think about it: You learn about all kinds of things that make life more enjoyable from your healthy friends. You learn about store

"Life is better . . . together."

Unknown author

sales, events, fun activities, and interesting people. Why leave diabetes out of the learning mix? Finding peers with diabetes, especially women, is very important to balance out your life. You can learn about new diabetes technology, tips for travel, deals on supplies, the locations of diabetes events, and much more.

Most of the first-time attendees at DiabetesSisters' Weekend for Women conferences report that they never knew another woman with diabetes prior to attending. Interestingly, 60% of people at the 2012 conference were repeat attendees. This speaks to the fact that women with diabetes crave a connection with other women who understand them, and once they find it, they will keep returning. Unfortunately, most women with diabetes live in isolation for far too long. When you consider that there are more than 246 million people worldwide (and 26 million people in the United States) living with diabetes, the idea of a person with diabetes not knowing another person with diabetes seems ludicrous. Yet, that is the reality for most people in the diabetes world. Diabetes is a "silent" disease that is easily and often tucked away.

DATING

Ahh . . . the fun years of dating! Can you sense my sarcasm? While this can be a fun time in a woman's life, for the woman with diabetes, it often sets off alarm bells. Some women feel that they bring a lot of baggage to the relationship. Others worry that men view them as less fertile. Others have even said that insulin pumps, scarred fingertips, and bad low blood sugar experiences in public have made them feel less sexy or confident in themselves.

As women, we think about everything *a lot.* My husband will tell you that women have a tendency to overthink things. But rather than trying to *stop* overthinking, I think we need to change the way we think. Again and again, I have met women who feel as though they are burdening men with their diabetes. And yet, I don't know a single man who is without a fault or problem of his own. Let's face it—we all have issues. Some are physical, some are psychological, some are spiritual, some are familial, and some are social. Make no mistake: The man you just talked to at that party or game, the one who seems so perfect, he has issues. It's just a matter of uncovering them. And isn't it better to get our issues out on the table early on? For example, you might learn that in addition to having a great personality and strapping good looks, the guy you're interested in has experienced episodes of depression in his life. Or maybe he was diagnosed with asthma as a child. Would you automatically walk away from him? Probably not. You know that neither of these things are his fault, and depression and asthma both can be managed with the right medications.

Now think about you and your diabetes. It's not your fault and it can be managed with the right medication, right? The big barrier you are feeling is really in *your* head.

You might be interested to learn that the topic of dating a person with diabetes is so commonplace now, there are articles devoted to it on dating websites. On Match.com, you can find an article entitled, "Dating a Diabetic." And the article was written by a woman who is dating a man with diabetes. It never ceases to amaze me how understanding so many women are when the men in their lives have "issues" or imperfections, yet when the women themselves are struggling, they view themselves as unworthy of love or happiness. "The more time I spend with Matt, the more I've come to think of him as a regular guy who surfs and wears hoodies and goes to work and plays poker. He just happens to be diabetic. Those are the cards he was dealt, but with Matt I know I've got a good hand, I don't plan on folding anytime soon." Her words sum up how a good life partner should view your diabetes—a regular person who just happens to have diabetes. If your partner views your diabetes differently, it may be time to consider the long-term viability of your relationship.

"When do I tell the person I'm dating that I have diabetes?" I get this question a lot, and I always give the following advice:

- Don't wait to tell or try to hide it. You don't have to bring it up on the first date, but it's also not fair to keep a health condition like diabetes from the person you're dating. Watching a date have a low blood sugar reaction and then not finding out the person has diabetes until you get to the hospital can be alarming. It's always best to talk about something like this during a stress-free moment when you are both focused on each other.

- Be honest. Putting it all on the table takes courage and confidence, but you'll be glad you did. No one wants to waste time with the wrong person. Also, be sure to allow your partner to ask questions without being defensive. Remember, the average American knows very little about diabetes and the little they know is often incorrect.

- Communicate regularly and openly. Don't just mention diabetes once and expect to never talk about it again. The more at ease you are in discussing diabetes, the more comfortable your partner will be. Think of and talk about your diabetes as if it is your second job or one of your friends.

- Learn together. The diabetes world is ever-changing, with new technology, research, programs, foods, products, and events. Attend conferences and/or workshops together. You will be amazed at how thankful your partner is to learn about diabetes because knowledge is empowering for them. When significant others feel uninformed about your disease, they feel helpless. It's great to have a solution as simple as education or knowledge.

- Make your significant other part of your diabetes team. This step happens over time. Just as it took years for you to learn the basics about diabetes, it will take your mate years as well. Teach him/her in small doses: how you test your blood sugar and what the range should be, how you determine what foods to eat at a meal, how much insulin is required for a meal or snack. Eventually, you might want to work up to your partner attending a doctor's appointment with you.

Dating is hard and diabetes certainly doesn't make it any easier. What I hate to see happen is women staying in bad relationships with people who do not support them or who are unwilling to make their health a priority. Unfortunately, due to their fear of rejection, women with diabetes sometimes overlook the telltale signs of a bad life partner. Such a person might: avoid the subject of diabetes or be uncomfortable talking about it; show no interest in learning about diabetes (how it is managed, how to help you in an emergency situation, what the future looks like); make you feel bad about having diabetes; be embarrassed by your diabetes (doesn't want you to tell others that you have diabetes; continually doesn't recognize or acknowledge symptoms of low blood sugar; makes derogatory comments/jokes about your diabetes).

You should never apologize for having diabetes. By doing this, you are teaching others to view the disease as an inconvenience. Remember, you teach others how to think about and act toward your diabetes through your words and actions.

SOUL-SEARCHING

How does the person you are currently dating stack up when you think about the telltale signs listed above? Can you (or would you want to) count on him/her to make your health a priority in their life?

_____

_____

_____

MARRIAGE

There is no doubt that diabetes will have some impact on your marriage. After all, it's a part of you. If diabetes doesn't have some impact on your marriage, it probably isn't being given enough attention in your relationship. The real question is how will diabetes affect your marriage? It's like pregnancy in that someone can tell you what it's like, but you never really know until you experience it for yourself. Each case is unique and individual.

Erratic Emotions

One thing that surprised my husband was the wide range of emotions that result from high and low blood sugars. When I am high or low, I can very quickly go from being a completely normal, lovable woman to, well, the exact opposite. For example, when I am low, I can be pretty impatient and mean, which is out of character for me. When my blood sugar is high, I am extremely tired and nauseated and just want to lie down. Lethargy is out of character for me as well. Most women with diabetes report similar experiences, though each woman has her own unique symptoms.

Such erratic emotions can put strain on your relationship with your spouse, so be prepared to address situations openly when they occur. It's always best to familiarize your spouse with your symptoms of high and low early on in the relationship. A willingness to apologize for your negative behavior is priceless in these situations.

Finances

There is no doubt that diabetes will cost you and your spouse money. It is an expensive disease, especially if you do not have health insurance. Having good health insurance drastically reduces the financial strain caused by diabetes. My husband is very healthy, so his health care costs are very small. However, between my diabetes medications, pump supplies, meter supplies, endocrinologist visits, ophthalmology visits, and lab tests, I can always be counted on to make us reach the insurance deductible. While this could cause conflict, my husband has never once made me feel bad about the costs associated with my diabetes. Instead, he says, "You know what you need to live. I don't. I just want you to take care of yourself so we can grow old together. The cost is not my concern." That's exactly why I love him!

However, if you do experience conflict over the financial burden of diabetes, you should know that you are not in the minority. Money is the most common cause of marital conflict among those who do not have diabetes, so you can imagine that this is amplified when a costly chronic illness is added to the marital mix.

Always be open and honest about the financial cost of diabetes and what can be expected, before you get married, so there are no surprises after the ceremony.

Underlying Feelings

Both you and your spouse will likely experience feelings of sadness, despair, anger, helplessness, and loss of control due to your diabetes at various times during your relationship. This is normal. Rather than letting the feelings fester, it's important for both you and your spouse to share them openly and honestly. Communicating rather than denying your feelings may help bring you closer. If the same feeling persists for either of you for more than 2 weeks, it may be time to make an appointment with your mental health provider. Remember, depression is more likely in people with diabetes, but it is prevalent in the general population as well.

Food/Nutrition

I have heard many women talk about not wanting to deny their families the foods they love by making them switch over to their healthy diets. But wait a minute, isn't healthy better? Yes, your husband or partner may enjoy meat and potatoes every day of the week and your child may enjoy sugary sweet cereal every morning of the week, but is that what is best for them? As the primary decision-makers when it comes to the health of our families (and in America, women generally do carry this responsibility more than men), we hold a lot more power than we give ourselves credit for. This is a great opportunity to change your perspective and help your entire family become healthier. It may be difficult at first to get buy-in from your family, but stick with it. They'll thank you in the end. By focusing on the value of healthy eating rather than the deficits inflicted by diabetes, everyone will have a more positive outlook.

Changing Plans

While no one wants diabetes to stop them from doing everything they want to do in life, there are times when it puts a cramp in

your daily plans. A high blood sugar or a low blood sugar may take you out of commission for a few hours, nixing or delaying the well-laid plans made by your spouse. Naturally, there is always a potential for this to create tension. Again, the key to success in this situation is for both partners to communicate their feelings openly and honestly. More often than not, you are just as frustrated as your partner and vice versa. This can bring you closer to each other.

Pregnancy/Family

Your partner likely has questions and concerns about your ability to carry a child. This is completely normal. Hopefully, all of these questions will be addressed long before the question of marriage comes about. Even if you decide to go through with pregnancy, there is still a great deal of attention that must be paid to your health in order to ensure a healthy baby and mom. These new requirements and increased attention to your diabetes can create its own set of tension. Decisions about whether or not to have more children may also be affected by your diabetes.

Sex

Whether it's frequent low blood sugars during sex, complications from diabetes that affect your arousal, or diabetes' effect on your ability to feel sexy, diabetes will have an impact on your sex life with your spouse at one time or another. Each couple's stress points are different, but it's good to think through them before you encounter them. It's also good to know that you are not alone.

SOUL-SEARCHING

What are some of the ways that diabetes has affected your marriage (positively and negatively)?

_____

_____

_____

LIFE APPLICATION

Invite your spouse/partner to manage your diabetes for a day or a weekend. This includes testing your blood sugar, making food choices, counting carbs, and doing medications. Yes, it will be hard to see him/her make a mistake in carb counting or medication dosing, but it is the best way for him/her to experience what you go through on a daily basis.

1. Ask your partner what surprised him/her about your daily diabetes management requirements?

   _____

   _____

   _____

2. Ask your spouse/partner how he/she thinks diabetes has positively and negatively affected your marriage. Record his/her answers below.

   _____

   _____

   _____

MY DIABETES JOURNAL

What was most surprising about your spouse's view of your diabetes and its impact on your marriage?

   _____

   _____

   _____

   _____

How did it feel to talk openly and honestly about your diabetes with your spouse?

_____

_____

_____

Did you uncover any other insightful information during your conversation?

_____

_____

_____

PARENTING/CHILDREN

If you are diagnosed with diabetes before the birth of your child or during your early years, diabetes will become a part of the child's "normal" way of life. As your children grow, they will see you doing all of the things you do to take care of yourself. This is what most mothers do, right? At some point, it will dawn on them that all moms don't have diabetes and they will probably become curious. Talk with them openly and candidly about your diabetes. Help them understand why you need to prick your finger or take a shot. Be positive. Your child's view of diabetes is greatly affected by your view of it. If you are frequently heard making statements such as, "I hate this disease. Diabetes ruined my life," they will hate the disease and see it as a burden. On the other hand, if they see you regularly checking your blood sugar, taking your insulin, exercising, eating healthily, and enjoying life, they will view diabetes more positively.

Of course, when they are really young they won't understand much beyond you "taking your medicine." But as they mature, they will be able to understand more and more. They may even want to get involved and help you by doing things like bringing something to treat a low, bringing you your testing kit, or pricking your finger.

When the time is right, you might consider talking with them about times where you really might need their help, such as if they should find you unconscious. Teaching them how to call for help is an important step. Practice dialing 9-1-1 without actually calling and practice what they should say to the emergency operator. It can be as simple as, "My name is_____. My address is _____. My mom has diabetes and needs help." Take them to a police station or fire station, and show them what a responding officer's uniform might look like, and explain that it is okay to unlock the door for them, especially when they have initiated a call to them. Teach them to inform the emergency responders about your diabetes. Consider making a "cheat sheet" that they can put somewhere in case they ever need it. Hopefully they'll never need to use it, but it's better for them to know what to do and not need it than to experience an emergency and not know.

Most people say that not knowing what to do in an emergency is the most intimidating aspect of being around a person with diabetes. So, eliminating this anxiety in your children, friends, and family will probably be very much appreciated. Depending on their age and maturity level, you may also introduce a glucagon kit to your children, and show them when/how to use it.

Even with the most positive outlook about diabetes, children will still worry about you. It's natural. One eye-opening moment occurred for me while I was conducting an impromptu video interview with my daughter, Summer, who was 7 at the time. I asked her if she worried about my diabetes, and her response stopped me dead in my tracks. She said, "Yeah, I worry about you being at home by yourself during the day working and having a low blood sugar with no one here to help you." I followed up by asking, "How often do you think about this?" She replied, "A few times every day. I think about it a lot while I'm at school." Of course, I had no idea that she was going through this mental anguish on a daily basis and while at school, when she was supposed to be learning, having fun with friends, and being a carefree second grader.

Unless circumstances dictate otherwise, it's best to let your kids control how much information they receive about diabetes, and how quickly, to avoid overwhelming them. Welcome questions and let them know that you will answer anything they want to know about diabetes. Be sure to answer any questions from your kids with a positive outlook. You'll be amazed how your positive outlook will have a lasting influence on your child and their thoughts about your disease.

As they get older, your children may ask whether they will develop diabetes. The true answer is that the odds of them developing diabetes are very slim (but not impossible). If your child has a positive view of you and your experience with diabetes, this will not be as anxiety-provoking. Still, you may worry about this possibility as you watch your kids grow up. When they are thirsty and drinking more than usual, you'll wonder if it could be diabetes, or is it just from playing outside on a hot summer day? When they wake to use the bathroom more than once in the night, you'll have that little question in the back of your head. That may never leave. It's just a part of being a concerned parent, who happens to have diabetes. The likelihood your child will develop diabetes is actually pretty low, though there is a stronger genetic link shown with type 2 diabetes than with type 1 diabetes. In type 2 diabetes, if you have a sibling or a parent who has the disease, your risk is as high as 1 in 3. And if you have two siblings or two parents who have the disease, it's higher still. According to Dr. James Warram of Harvard University School of Public Health, the risk for a child of a parent with type 1 diabetes is lower if it is the mother—rather than the father—who has diabetes. If the father has it, the risk is about 1 in 10 (10%) that his child will develop type 1 diabetes—the same as the risk to a sibling of an affected child. On the other hand, if the mother has type 1 diabetes and is age 25 or younger when the child is born, the risk is reduced to 1 in 25 (4%) and if the mother is over age 25, the risk drops to 1 in 100—virtually the same as the average American.

Remember, your first and most important duty as a parent is to keep yourself healthy so you can care for your family. As a woman, you will often be torn in many different directions with various family demands, but it is important for you to serve as a good role model for your children and family by outwardly making your health a top priority. Your mental health is an important part of your overall health, so don't ignore symptoms of hopelessness, helplessness, sadness, or being overwhelmed that last more than 2 weeks. Reach out to a mental health care provider or a physician. The challenges of diabetes management on top of those associated with motherhood can easily overwhelm a woman. It happens a lot more often than you think.

SOUL-SEARCHING

What messages (positive and negative) have you sent your child about diabetes? How did you send these messages? (Verbally, through your behavior, etc.)

_____

_____

_____

LIFE APPLICATION

Talk to your children about your diabetes. Ask them if they have any questions about your diabetes. Then, depending on their ages, you might ask some questions of your own, though not all at the same time. Is diabetes good or bad? What are your thoughts about people who have diabetes? Do you worry about my diabetes? What concerns you? Do you know what to do if I have a low blood sugar? Do you know the symptoms to look for?

MY DIABETES JOURNAL

What did you uncover about your child's view of diabetes? Where could you help improve their understanding or view of the disease? What is the main message you want to convey to your children about living with diabetes? What is the best way to do this?

_____

_____

_____

_____

_____

EXTENDED FAMILY

Most people have at least one member of the "diabetes police squad" among their extended family members. Family gatherings are usually where we see and hear them. These are the family members who make the dreaded comments aimed at you, like, "You can't have that, can you?" or "You're not supposed to eat sweets!" They're also the ones who are full of judgment because they don't understand why we just can't manage our diabetes. After all, it would be easy for them, right?

Most of the time, these are well-intentioned family members who are truly uneducated about diabetes. Unknowingly, they are members of the "diabetes police squad." It's easy to be insulted and hurt by their words. However, these experiences can be great educational experiences for the entire family. I can recall one experience where a family member did just what was described above, and I had a quick reply ready. "Of course I can eat this. I take good care of my diabetes . . . and I counted for it in my insulin bolus." What ensued was an insightful conversation with a few family members about diabetes management goals. Again, just as with significant others and spouses, open and honest communication is key.

SOUL-SEARCHING

Who are the "diabetes police" in your family? What are some of the most hurtful things said/done to you by them?

_____

_____

_____

_____

_____

LIFE APPLICATION

Talk with at least one family member you have identified as a member of the "diabetes police." Ask him/her what he/she knows about diabetes. Ask what his/her biggest fear/concern is about your diabetes. Ask who else he/she knows who has diabetes, and what that person's experience was with diabetes. Develop a well thought-out plan for responding to family members' intrusive comments.

_____

_____

_____

_____

_____

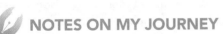

MY DIABETES JOURNAL

What did you uncover about your family member's view of diabetes? How was this conversation different from previous conversations with him/her about diabetes?

_____

_____

_____

_____

What did you discover about yourself through this exercise?

_____

_____

_____

_____

_____

_____

NOTES ON MY JOURNEY

_____

_____

_____

_____

TIPS FOR FRIENDS AND FAMILY MEMBERS OF WOMEN WITH DIABETES

- Respect the amount of work and attention that goes into managing diabetes, on top of all of the other things she must do in her life. When there is an opportunity to verbally recognize her hard work, do so.
- Do not be judgmental. Recognize that you likely could not manage diabetes better than she does, and even if, by chance, you could, it would do no good to voice this thought.
- Praise her for the strength and courage she shows in managing a lifelong, 24-hour-a-day chronic illness.
- Allow her to have emotional moments of desperation, anger, sorrow, and weakness regarding her diabetes. No one can be strong all the time.
- Be flexible. Never show anger when a high or low blood sugar causes you an inconvenience or change of plans.
- Allow her to be the diabetes expert. Learn from her. You do not know more than her about her diabetes.
- Never assume that the things you have heard on television or read on the Internet about diabetes are true. Ask her for clarification about anything you find confusing.
- Understand very clearly that no one caused their own diabetes and no one wants to have the disease. There are many factors that contribute to a diagnosis of type 2 diabetes, only one of which is weight. Others factors include family history, high cholesterol, high blood pressure, age, race/ethnic background, and history of gestational diabetes. No one knows what causes type 1 diabetes.
- She may secretly feel less "pretty" or less "desirable" because of her diabetes. Whenever you have the chance to compliment her beauty, please do.
- Read as much information about diabetes from reputable medical sources as possible.

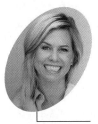

Travel

NATALIE SAYS...

Traveling with diabetes can be a challenge. As many of you may know, I competed in and won an adventure travel reality show called *The Amazing Race*. In this competition, teams of two race around the world, completing a series of physical, intellectual, and logistical challenges with nothing but a backpack. I traveled over 32,000 miles with no money, no cell phone, no guide book, and no plans. Everything for an entire month had to fit in one pack, including clothing suitable for deserts and for the Arctic Circle. I had no idea about a schedule. I had no ability to plan meals ahead. Anyone would have a tough time with this, but add packing for type 1 diabetes and dealing with diabetes on the road, and you have a real challenge!

Let me tell you about a conversation I had with my diabetes educator one month before I went on *The Amazing Race*. I called Carolyn and said, "I'm going to do this reality travel show where I travel around the world, visit a new country every day, run, hike, climb, swim, eat irregular meals, have lots of stress, and no communication with you or anyone else. Oh yeah, and I only

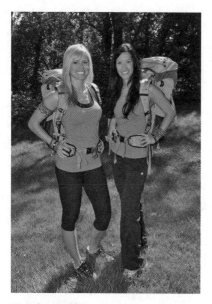

Natalie and her teammate, Kat, compete and win *The Amazing Race*. *CBS via Getty Images.*

have one backpack to squeeze everything into. Now what?" I always knew that I would do the race, but working with Carolyn helped me figure out how.

I couldn't believe how helpful she was. I was really impressed with not only the depth of her knowledge, but also with the vast array of life issues that she helped me to anticipate. We planned for highs, lows, pump failures, the confiscation of supplies by customs officials, heat, cold, jet lag, and dehydration. It was her idea to type up a letter of medical necessity in every language we could think of explaining why I needed these syringes and vials. That way I could travel in remote parts of the world and be able to explain why I was traveling with a mini pharmacy in my backpack. It was Carolyn who told me how I could use a Frio pouch to keep my insulin cold without ice or refrigeration. She helped me figure out a way to repackage my pump supplies so they would take up less room in my backpack. She convinced Medtronic to give me a loaner insulin pump in case mine got wet or compromised. She drew upon her experience with thousands of patients to imagine every complication and solution she could think of. We knew the speed bumps were inevitable, but we also knew that with good preparation nothing was going to be impossible.

Not only did I complete the entire *Amazing Race* experience free of any diabetes-related complications, but my teammate, Kat, and I won! We became the first female team to win in *Amazing Race* history, and I did it with diabetes.

So I know firsthand how complicated traveling with diabetes can be. Supplies, meals, exercise, time zone changes, it can all

"Twenty years from now you will be more disappointed
by the things that you didn't do than by the ones you did
do. So throw off the bowlines. Sail away from the safe
harbor. Catch the trade winds in your sails. Explore.
Dream. Discover."

Unknown

affect our blood sugar management. But I firmly believe that we
can all travel safely and that we should!

Whether you are getting ready for your inner Indiana Jones
to come out while you zip-line through South America or you
are getting ready to go to Aunt Nellie's wedding in Nebraska,
planning ahead can ensure you have a safe and fun experience.
Let me say this again: Planning ahead is *the* most important thing
you can do to make your travels worry-free. It's so important for
me to get the message out there that anything and *everything* is
possible with diabetes. It breaks my heart when women with
diabetes skip out on things because they think that their diabetes
makes it impossible for them. I know marathoners who have
run across the Sahara Desert, hikers who have climbed Mt. Everest, and race car drivers who have raced all around the world …
with diabetes.

ONE MONTH BEFORE YOUR TRIP

One month in advance may seem very early to begin prepping
for your trip, but for abroad trips or remote locations, this will
definitely work to your advantage! You don't want to wait until
the day before and then be frantically trying to reach your doctor
for a prescription refill! It's a great idea to see your physician
weeks in advance of your trip, especially if you might need vaccines. Make sure you have all of your prescriptions up to date,
and perhaps extra amounts of medication to avert disaster if you
lose a purse, drop an insulin vial, or get food poisoning and toss
your pills along with your cookies. Also, this is the time to make

sure that your medical alert bracelet is up to date (or buy one if you still don't have one). It's also a good time to talk to your physician about any activities that you may be planning, both to make sure your health is optimized and also to strategize for working with your diabetes to do any activity safely. *Anything and everything* is possible with diabetes, but it may take some advance planning. Work with your physician to scuba dive safely (I reduce my basal rate when diving to avoid hypoglycemia and also bring a waterproof sugar source with me so I can treat below the surface if needed). Plan out an insulin or medication reduction if you are doing an active trip like skiing or surfing.

This is also an opportunity to get a letter from your physician to help you navigate security safely. If you travel with juice to treat low blood sugars, having a prescription signed by your doctor that says you have diabetes and that the juice is needed for medical purposes will help. I will go into going through security later in the chapter, but that can be an adventure in itself!

If you are traveling to a country where you don't speak the language, I find it helpful to use an online translator to type out a letter in the local language that explains that you have diabetes, what your medications are for, and your emergency contact information. I also make it a personal goal to learn how to say, "I have diabetes," "I need sugar," and "thanks" in every language I can.

For a fun challenge, try learning how to say "I have diabetes" in the following languages:

French: J'ai le diabète

Spanish: Tengo diabetes

Italian: Ho il diabete

Chinese: 我有糖尿病 (This one I just print out on a note!)

Depending on the length of your trip, this is also the time to get to know the local medical care. For example, when I studied abroad in France for 6 months in college, I didn't come home for endocrinology visits and refills. Instead, I located an English-speaking physician and established care in my new location. It was problem-free, and I had someone local in case of emergency (I was fine though).

There are several resources for locating medical care while traveling abroad. The quality of drugs and medical products abroad can't really be guaranteed, so bring all medications that you will need with you from home. This includes pain relievers and anti-diarrheal medication. Make sure to bring your own injection supplies, and if you do require an injection abroad, insist that a new needle and syringe be used.

According to the Centers for Disease Control and Prevention, the following resources list health care providers and facilities around the world:

- The Department of State (www.usembassy.gov) can help travelers locate medical services and notify friends, family, or employers about emergencies

- The International Society of Travel Medicine (ISTM) maintains a directory of health care professionals with expertise in travel medicine in almost 50 countries worldwide. Search these clinics at www.istm.org

- The International Association for Medical Assistance to Travelers (IAMAT) maintains an international network of physicians, hospitals, and clinics that have agreed to provide care to members while abroad. Membership is free, although donations are suggested. Search for clinics at http://www.iamat.org/doctors_clinics.cfm

- The Joint Commission International (JCI) aims to improve patient safety through accreditation and certification of health care facilities worldwide. Facilities that are accredited through JCI demonstrate a standard level of quality. A list of these facilities can be found at http://www.jointcommissioninternational.org/JCI-Accredited-Organizations

- Embassies and consulates in other countries, hotel doctors, and credit card companies (especially those with special privileges) may also provide useful information

- Supplemental medical insurance plans acquired prior to travel will often enable access to local health care providers in many countries through 24-hour emergency hotlines

I also think that it is wise for travelers with diabetes, or any chronic health condition, to purchase trip cancellation insurance for big trips. I normally ignore that kind of stuff (travel fees are expensive enough as it is!) but if you need to postpone or cancel a trip because you are ill, this will protect some or all of your financial investment. Expect the unexpected!

If you are going to be doing a lot of walking, this is a great time to purchase a new pair of shoes and comfortable clothing for exercise. You don't want to be breaking in a new pair of walking shoes on the first day of your trip. Blisters can ruin a trip for anyone, but for those of us with diabetes, it's extra important to avoid trauma to our feet. Get a pair of comfortable walking shoes and break them in before you go on vacation. Make sure that you have appropriate clothing as well. Loose-fitting, moisture-wicking clothing is best if you are going to work up a sweat.

KEY POINTS:

- See your health care provider
- Plan out medication changes for activities like walking, skiing, surfing, etc.
- Fill prescriptions/have extra amounts of everything. I take double what I think I will need
- Purchase any necessary travel supplies (insulation cases, diabetes organizers, new shoes, etc.)
- Make sure you have a medical alert bracelet or necklace that is up to date. Order one if you don't have one.
- Know the names of all of your medical conditions, your allergies, and your medications and print these out in the local language. Try to learn how to say them in the local language if possible.

ONE WEEK BEFORE YOUR TRIP

You have seen your physician, picked up any prescriptions that you needed, and ordered any new diabetes gadgets that are going to make your trip easier. Good job! One week before your trip is a great time to start preparing what you are going to pack and purchase any last-minute items. This is when I fill up on my snacks to treat low blood sugars, things such as Shot Bloks and Sport Beans. I like these because they replenish electrolytes as well, so if I am being active, they will help out with more than just the blood glucose level. They also don't melt, they are compact, and the packaging is waterproof. Whatever it is you will be doing, make sure that your glucose source is something that will be convenient. Take into account the temperature of your travel destination, where you will be carrying your glucose/snacks/medications, etc.

This is also a great time to think about how you are going to carry your medications and/or supplies around. While a giant purse is my travel case of choice most days, with lots of walking, that bag is going to get heavy very quickly! I recommend getting a good backpack. This is good for traveling; it will fit your medications, your water bottle (that you can fill *after* you go through security), your books, and your diabetes supplies. It will be easy to carry. It will also prevent you from leaving things behind, thinking, "I won't need that." I always carry a set of everything I'll need and one backup at all times. You never know when you will need something, and Murphy's Law always kicks in on vacation: If you carry everything on you, you won't need it.

I remember one trip to Belize when I was a teenager. I was going through a cave that had recently been filmed by National Geographic. It was over 2 miles deep into a mountainside, and filled with beautiful paintings and pots left by Mayan Indians. However, I didn't have that many diabetes supplies on me; I only had one small case of glucose. I worried the whole time about what would happen if I got low and ate all of my glucose. Then what? I was fine, but it definitely took away from the experience.

If I had packed a backpack with more than enough of everything I would need, I definitely could have relaxed more and enjoyed my adventure!

Alternatives to a backpack include hip packs (also known as fanny packs) and cross-body travel purses. I think it's helpful to make sure that whatever it is you will be carrying can zip shut so supplies won't spill out. A couple small pockets on the exterior of the bag allows for easy access to blood glucometers, medications, or glucose.

Now, being prepared doesn't have to mean schlepping a gigantic bag around. There are some space-saving techniques you can use. If you use test strips to monitor your blood sugar, you can put strips of the same company and same code in the same bottle. I've found that most test strip bottles will hold two times the amount of test strips that they usually come with. If you take oral medications, pill organizers can come in handy, keep a week's worth of medications organized, and save space at the same time. Always bring the original containers, though: They may be important. When organizing diabetes supplies, don't be afraid to get creative. While there are several good organizers out there, I actually prefer to use makeup cases. I get large ones with several compartments, then I have my insulin compartment where I put syringes, alcohol swabs, pump supplies, etc. I then have my blood glucose testing compartments where I have my test strips, lancets, backup meter, continuous glucose monitoring supplies, etc. I find the waterproof and clear exteriors of these bags make it easy to stay organized. Plus, you can pick them up in any pharmacy or drugstore, so it's great if you have some last-minute organizing to do!

A very important packing tip to remember is to always have diabetes supplies in two locations. Do not make the mistake of putting your supplies in your suitcase with only a day's worth of materials in your carry-on bag. Bags get lost! I always have a full set in my suitcase and in my carry-on bag. I also now use hard-cased carry-on bags. They make me feel more secure, knowing my supplies are protected.

KEY POINTS:

- Gather your glucose supplies and snacks, taking at least twice as much as you think you need
- Start packing your diabetes pack. Choose a backpack, hip sack, or purse that has a zipper and multiple side pockets for easy access
- Get a pill organizer and fill it with your medications
- Have a full set of supplies packed in your carry-on and in your checked luggage

LIFE APPLICATION

Make a checklist of all of your diabetes-related supplies and medications that you use in a week. Write it down here. Refer to this when packing to make sure you don't forget anything!

_____   _____

_____   _____

_____   _____

_____   _____

_____   _____

_____   _____

_____   _____

_____   _____

Natalie's List (for reference):

1. Insulin Delivery
   a. Insulin
   b. Syringes
   c. Alcohol swabs
   d. Insulin pump reservoirs and infusion sets
   e. Insulin storage/cooling
   f. Long- and short-acting insulins (in case pump fails for some reason)
   g. Batteries for pump

2. Blood Glucose Monitoring
   a. Test strips
   b. Meter ×2 (I always bring an extra one)
   c. Lancets
   d. Continuous glucose monitor (CGM) and transmitter
   e. CGM sensor (double the estimated need)
   f. CGM charger

3. Hypoglycemia Treatments
   a. Glucose tablets, Shot Bloks, Sport Beans
   b. Glucose gel
   c. Glucagon shot
   d. Carbohydrate snacks
   e. Carrier for these during exercise (arm bands, etc.)

4. Paperwork
   a. Letter of medical necessity, in local language if necessary
   b. Copies of prescriptions
   c. Medical Alert ID
   d. Travel insurance/local medical facilities resources

Once you have decided on your type of vacation, it's time to start thinking about all the things that may affect your diabetes and start finding your solutions. Here are some common scenarios and some solutions to challenges that these may present.

- Trips to warm-weather destinations
- Trips to cold-weather destinations
- Trips involving water sports, like playing in the pool or snorkeling
- Trips that involve a lot of walking or other exercise
- Trips to countries where you don't speak the language
- Trips to remote locations
- Trips to places with unfamiliar foods

TRIPS INVOLVING WARM WEATHER

Congratulations! You've just booked your trip to Mexico/Arizona/ Florida! Let's think about how you can prepare for this. The first thing that comes to my mind is, how are you going to keep insulin or other medications cold? Hopefully your accommodations will be able to offer you a refrigerator.

You will also need to be able to keep your insulin cold while you are on the go. There are many options for medication-carrying pouches that are insulated, have ice packs in them, or are water-activated to keep cold. These can be used to keep your medications safe and organized while traveling and also while you enjoy the beach/boat/golf course. You may also want to think about what healthy snacks you can travel with that won't be messy if they melt.

Another thing to consider is that with heat comes sweat, and it's more difficult keeping adhesives on your skin. This applies to insulin pumps and continuous glucose monitors. Be sure to check your stock and make sure you have two to three times the amount of these products that you normally would use. You also may dress differently at the beach than you do at home. If you normally wear your insulin pump in your jacket or pants pockets, you may need to get creative when you are in a bikini or sundress. This is a good time to shop around for products that carry your pump or keep it safe. Ideas include leg wraps, armbands, and belts.

Lastly, remember to drink plenty of water. Dehydration is hazardous for anyone, but even more so for those of us living with diabetes. You may want to bring a reusable water bottle with you to make sure you don't stop drinking water just because you are on the road.

TRIPS INVOLVING COLD WEATHER

Now let's pretend we are leaving our home in sunny California for a trip to Colorado in February. We still need to keep insulin away from extremes of temperature. This means not leaving it by a heater once we return inside from the cold outdoors. When things get really chilly, it's possible for our glucose meters to get so cold that they won't work. Try to keep them in a warm place, such as an inner pocket on a cardigan, when you are doing outdoor activities.

Also, remember that it can be difficult to test your blood glucose if your hands are really cold and your vessels are all constricted. Make sure to keep your hands warm, or at least warm them up and get your blood flowing before you test your blood sugar.

TRIPS INVOLVING WATER SPORTS

These are my favorite kinds of trips, but they are also some of the more challenging when it comes to diabetes. I love to snorkel, scuba dive, and swim in the pool and ocean ... but these are all scenarios that make it difficult to test your blood sugar and to keep your supplies dry. This also may be a challenge for those of us who use insulin pumps to manage our diabetes. Please check with your endocrinologist and your pump manufacturer about the safety of using your device in the water. Some pumps are waterproof, and others aren't. It may be necessary to detach from the pump for a short period of time. It may also be an option to use injectable insulin for a few days if your doctor thinks it is safe. Keep in mind, even if you have a waterproof pump as I do, play-ing in pools, putting on scuba equipment, etc., may all lead to accidental pump detachment. Have extra pump supplies and keep them with you!

Water sports also make treating a low blood sugar interesting. If you are in water, glucose tablets are likely to be messy or difficult to use. I like to have something that is sealed, and easy to ingest. Options include glucose gels and Sport Beans. I have a friend who tucks a package of Shot Bloks in her wetsuit when she goes surfing. Getting creative can ensure that you can safely pursue water sports!

TRIPS THAT INVOLVE A LOT OF WALKING

Many people enjoy vacations that involve a lot of walking. This is great! However, if your normal life involves sitting at a desk or in a car most of the day, this may mean some adjustments need to be made. Speak to your doctor about your trip. Estimate the number of hours per day you will be walking. You may need to decrease your insulin-to-carb ratio, or change some of your medications. We often underestimate the amount of exercise we are getting, wandering from sight to sight while on vacation. Also, make sure to always have some fast-acting sugar on hand. You don't want to be in an unfamiliar territory, looking for the nearest café or pharmacy. It's also a good idea to increase the frequency of your blood glucose testing. With all of the variables that accompany travel, like time zone changes, fatigue, excitement, food changes, and increased activity, it's important to know what your blood sugar is doing and what trends are developing.

It's also important to have good walking shoes. The shoes should be comfortable, worn-in, and have a good fit to avoid blisters and other injuries to our feet. When shopping for shoes, make sure you do so at the end of the day, when your feet may be a little more swollen. Also, get shoes with a big toe box, the area at the very front of the shoe. Stylish pointy shoes, even if they are flats, may become your worst enemy if you develop blisters. If you are buying new shoes, make sure you break them in at home before you go on your vacation. Also, be prepared. Have moleskin, band-aids, and antibacterial ointment on hand just in case a blister does develop.

TRIPS TO FOREIGN COUNTRIES

I love traveling to new and foreign places, but to be safe, there are a few precautions that I always take. I always recommend carrying a letter that explains your diabetes, that lists your medications and your allergies, and that lists your emergency contact information. Have this letter in English and in the language of the country that you are visiting. Let's hope you never need it, but it could be the difference between an adventure and a disaster. Also, if you can, try to learn how to say a few key phrases in the local language. I try to at least learn the following:

"Hello. Can you help me? I have diabetes. I need sugar. Thank you."

This can be useful in restaurants, with locals, and it's always helpful to be able to thank kind strangers! When I was traveling through Egypt once, I was in a long taxi ride and I needed to stop and get some food. I told the taxi driver that I needed sugar, and he stopped at a café. It made me feel comfortable to know that I could communicate my needs to someone, even if they didn't know English. Don't worry; even if you don't want to learn a new phrase, just having it written out on a piece of paper that you keep in your wallet can help.

TRAVELING TO REMOTE LOCATIONS

Many of the world's most beautiful places are remote and not filled with pharmacies. That's what makes them so appealing. However, if you are someone who uses medication on a daily basis for diabetes, blood pressure, heart conditions, asthma, etc., it can be intimidating to explore these remote locations. Under your physician's care, it can be safely done, however, and I encourage everyone to try it! It just takes some planning to make sure you avoid any problems.

Be sure to take at least double the amount of medication you think you will need. If some gets lost, falls into a toilet, or is stolen, you want to be prepared. This also means having your medication in more than one location. Have a full supply in your purse or backpack when traveling. Have another full supply in your luggage. If you are traveling with a spouse or a friend, ask them to also carry some medication for you. This way, you are safeguarding against ever running out, or losing access to your medication. Also, make sure you have glucagon, glucose gels, and other hypoglycemic treatments readily available. Make sure your travel mates know where this is located *and* how to use it. Trips to adventurous places are always a great time to refresh your friends and family on how to treat a severe low blood sugar.

There are other considerations besides medication. These include batteries for your insulin pump, blood glucose meter, or other medical devices. Have these with you; it's not guaranteed that you will find batteries when you need them, even in tourist areas. Also make sure that you have the appropriate conversion tools to be able to plug in any rechargeable devices you may have like continuous glucose monitors.

TRIPS INVOLVING UNFAMILIAR FOODS

Sampling the local cuisine is a large part of exploring new areas. Even if you are not going far from home, your usual meals are likely to be altered with frequent dining out at restaurants. If you will have access to a kitchen during your travels, you are lucky. Stopping by a grocery store once you reach your destination will allow you to purchase some of your familiar foods so you can maintain some normalcy. I often will purchase supplies for snacks and light meals. If eating out will be a large part of your vacation, try to make smart choices. Educate yourself on the local fare before you leave on your trip. Are you dying to eat couscous in Morocco? Take a look at the carbohydrate count in an average serving so you have an idea of what to expect when you get there. Another tactic is to base your meal primarily on proteins and vegetables, and save the high carbohydrate dish as a side order. This way, even if your estimates for that mouth-watering risotto in Italy are off, it's a smaller portion so the margin of error is likely to be smaller. As always, increase the frequency of your blood sugar monitoring. You don't want to be guessing! Testing 2 hours after a meal is an excellent way to determine if you were over or under estimating the carbohydrates and insulin requirements.

🔍 SOUL-SEARCHING

Have you passed up on any trips because of your diabetes? If so, what, in particular, about your diabetes held you back?

_____

_____

_____

_____

Have you noticed that your diabetes is more difficult to control when you travel? If so, look back on a recent trip and see if you can identify three things in particular that affected your diabetes.

1. _____

2. _____

3. _____

In the future, what strategies can you use to address these three things when you travel?

_____

_____

_____

_____

_____

_____

_____

_____

_____

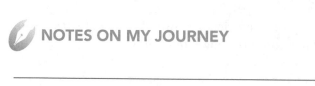 **NOTES ON MY JOURNEY**

_____

_____

_____

_____

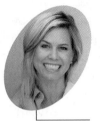

Exercise

NATALIE SAYS...

This is a very easy chapter for me to write because there are very few things I believe in more than exercise in terms of improving the quality of our lives with diabetes. If there was ever a miracle for people with diabetes, exercise is it! No matter where you are on the athletic spectrum, the fact that you are reading this chapter lets me know that you are on your way to a fitter, healthier, happier version of yourself. Hopefully, by the end of this chapter you'll have some new tips and tricks to apply to your own exercise routine.

In this section, I will cover everything I can think of related to exercise. I will go over the physiology of exercise and explain exactly how it works to make our bodies healthier. I'll talk about some of the common barriers to starting an exercise routine and go over strategies to help you make exercise part of your everyday life. I will discuss aspects of exercise that are particular to type 2 diabetes, and I will also talk about exercise as it relates to type 1 diabetes. With type 1 diabetes, I really want to address the idea that even though exercise can initially send us on a wild blood glucose chase, it's still definitely as important for us to exercise as it is for our type 2 sisters. I even want to talk about what to wear; feeling cute is important along with keeping our diabetes needs in mind.

Let's start with the basics. What exactly is exercise? Exercise is an activity requiring physical effort that is carried out to sustain or improve health and fitness. Anything that increases your activity level over your baseline qualifies as exercise in my book. This might mean getting out of your chair more at work. It might involve walking around the block when you get home. It can be gardening, biking, running, or even shopping. If you are moving more than normal, congratulations, you are exercising!

There are three main types of exercise: strength training, flexibility, and aerobic exercise. Strength training is not only for men, nor is it only for professional athletes. Every single woman with diabetes should be working with strength training. The American Diabetes Association currently recommends that we focus on strength training at least two times a week. Wondering why you should lift weights if you aren't concerned with bulging biceps? Consider this. Weightlifting can increase your muscle mass, which in turn increases your metabolism. This means you can continue to burn more calories long after the workout is finished. In addition, it can improve your insulin sensitivity. As women, we often find it harder to lose weight as we age because our metabolism slows down. Ever notice that our male counterparts have an easier time losing weight than we do? Well, women tend to lose muscle mass at almost twice the rate as men! Muscle is way more metabolically active than fat, so the more muscle we have, the more our metabolism jumps up. The more muscle we lose, the more our metabolism slows down. So, if you want to fight the metabolism decrease, you have to build muscle.

In addition to increasing our metabolism, strength training has a variety of diabetes-specific benefits as well. Studies have shown that weightlifting can increase bone density by as much as 3–5% per year! Increasing our bone density is important because, as women with diabetes, we are at a higher risk for osteoporosis. Having nice strong bones means that if we do have an accident or fall, we are not as likely to break a bone or get a fracture. In addition, studies have demonstrated benefits of strength training on our blood glucose levels, glucose tolerance, and insulin sensitivity. In one study of 40 women who did strength training three times a week for 4 months, the average A1C levels dropped from 8.7 to 7.6, the amount of diabetes medications decreased in 72% of the participants, and blood pressure dropped by 10 mmHg. Decreasing blood pressure is good news for our hearts and our kidneys, meaning a decreased risk for heart attacks, stroke, and kidney failure. Now, that's a reason to start a strength-training program!

Don't be intimidated; this doesn't have to mean lifting barbells in a gym full of muscle heads. You can use weights at home or even resistance bands. Just remember to discuss any new exercise with your doctor before you start and consider using a trainer or DVD to guide you if you are just beginning. You don't want to injure yourself!

Flexibility exercises are also important. As discussed in the chapter on physical health, living with diabetes does mean that we are at risk for changes in our muscles and ligaments. We are prone to losing range of motion and developing stiffness with conditions like frozen shoulder syndrome and stiff hand syndrome. In addition, glycosylation of joint structures in general (binding of glucose where it shouldn't bind) can also lead to decreased mobility in other locations like our lumbar spine. Taking time to stretch is very important to minimize the effects of diabetes on our musculoskeletal system and also to prevent injury associated with exercise. When we stretch we help maintain normal joint function by preserving mobility and flexibility. Stretching is also recommended as part of the warm-up and cool-down that's part of either strength exercises or aerobic exercise. Flexibility exercise includes pilates, yoga, or any stretching regimen. Correct stretching should be done after a warm-up period. You don't want to injure "cold" muscles. Do some mild aerobic activity for about 5 minutes to get your blood flowing before you start to stretch your muscles. Most experts currently recommend dynamic stretching before exercise, avoiding the static stretches that we were often taught in physical education classes. Dynamic stretching involves slow, controlled movements rather than remaining still and holding a stretch. This includes things like arm circles, hip rotations, or flowing movements like in yoga. Static stretches are more useful after your workout. This is a chance to lengthen muscles and improve flexibility; hold these stretches for about 30 seconds. Remember, stretching should never be painful. If you are making a face or holding your breath, back off a little bit. You should be able to relax into your stretch.

Aerobic exercise is probably the type of exercise that we are most familiar with, and with good reason. Aerobic exercise includes things like walking, running, biking, hiking, swimming, dancing, etc. Aerobic exercise uses oxygen to meet energy demands—hence the name aerobic, which means "in the air." We also commonly call this exercise cardio, short for cardiovascular exercise, since this exercise strengthens the heart and improves the resting heart rate and pumping efficiency. It improves circulation. It improves blood pressure. It increases oxygen transportation through the body. This is important because the microvascular complications of diabetes result in the tiny blood vessels that deliver oxygen to our tissues becoming blocked at times. Aerobic exercise also increases insulin sensitivity. Insulin sensitivity is how sensitive your body is to the effects of insulin. If you are insulin-resistant, your body experiences a smaller effect from insulin. If you are more insulin-sensitive, you have more of a response to insulin than if you are insulin-resistant. Aerobic exercise increases insulin sensitivity by increasing the uptake of glucose into the cells and moving it out of the bloodstream. This can allow people to reduce diabetes medications, or even eliminate them. It's important to know that this positive effect happens regardless of weight loss, although that can improve your sensitivity to insulin, too. One study found that aerobic exercise improved whole body insulin sensitivity by 40%.

Aerobic exercise improves glucose metabolism, too. Glucose transporters, which allow glucose to pass from the bloodstream into muscle cells, increase with exercise. This basically turns the glucose road from a one-lane road to a six-lane superhighway, letting our glucose get to where we want it to be ... out of our bloodstream and into the muscles. You can now see why exercise is such a gift for those of us with diabetes. Current recommendations for aerobic exercise are to get 30 minutes most days of the week for a total of 150–175 minutes per week. I know it sounds like a lot at first, but it is important to make this a part of your routine. It needs to be as important as your appointments, your deadlines, and your family's needs. Exercise is not something to fit into your day if you have the time.

Now that we have gone over the different types of exercise and why each type of exercise is important, let's talk about exercise in general and the positive effects it has on our diabetes and our bodies. Some of these have already been mentioned, but it never hurts to point out the goodness again!

Exercise:
- improves your body's ability to use insulin
- improves glucose metabolism
- helps with weight loss
- increases muscle strength
- increases metabolism (helps you burn more calories at rest)
- decreases blood pressure
- improves cholesterol
- improves blood flow
- decreases risk of heart disease
- decreases risk of stroke
- decreases risk of kidney failure
- increases energy
- improves moods and helps fight off or treat depression
- decreases anxiety
- improves sleep
- improves libido
- increases the function of your immune system
- fights osteoporosis

That is quite an impressive list. Some of you may have been surprised to see so many psychological benefits on there. Improved mood? Improved sleep? Decreased anxiety? Let's get into it. Exercise stimulates the production of serotonin and brain-derived neurotrophic factor (BDNF). Serotonin is commonly known as the "feel good" neurotransmitter. In fact, many anti-depressant medications work by increasing the amount of serotonin that our neurons are exposed to.

This is especially important because some sources state up to one in four women with diabetes will experience depression in their lifetime. Many women don't know it, but they try to give themselves serotonin boosts by snacking on sweets. Ever been prone to emotional eating? Ever feel like that bar of chocolate just makes you feel better? Well, carbohydrates can lead to a boost in serotonin. When you consume carbohydrates, neurotransmitters are signaled to release more serotonin and this makes us feel better. When we eat carbohydrates, we allow tryptophan to get into the brain. Since serotonin is made from tryptophan, our serotonin levels increase and we begin to feel better. Since exercise helps elevate our serotonin, we may be able to shift our self-medication with food to using exercise instead. Since sleep is also related to serotonin, our sleep improves with exercise as well. This also benefits our overall mood.

Exercise also blunts our response to stress and anxiety. When we get our heart rate up, we are stimulating our sympathetic nervous system, commonly referred to as the fight or flight response. Our body senses many of the same symptoms that occur with anxiety: rapid breathing, fast heart rate, sweating. With repeated exposures to these symptoms, the body becomes less and less reactive to them. This translates into your everyday life where stressors may trigger these physical responses, so the overall anxiety level and "fear response" is decreased. Studies have shown that anxiety levels are measurably decreased after only 2 weeks of regular exercise.

Exercise can also help us feel good by releasing endorphins. Endorphins are our body's natural pain relievers. They are made in the body and bind to opiate receptors in the nervous system to reduce our perception of pain, working in the same way that morphine does. In addition to a decrease in pain perception, endorphins also promote a sense of euphoria or well-being. This is what people are referring to when they describe a "runner's high." Strenuous exercise of any kind can lead to this, not only running.

Exercise can also help us control our diabetes by decreasing our appetite. Serotonin increases can decrease our appetite by promoting satiety, or a feeling of fullness.

So, what does all this serotonin stuff mean for us women with diabetes? It is very good news. Both diabetes and being a woman put us at an increased risk for depression, so add those together and you really have to pay attention. Exercise is at least as effective as antidepressants at treating depression. But what if you are just in a bad mood? It still helps. As little as 5 minutes of exercise can acutely improve mood! So next time you want a carbohydrate-rich snack, try taking a walk around the block instead and take note of what happens.

EXERCISE AND TYPE 1 DIABETES

There are several extra considerations for exercise if you are living with type 1 diabetes. In fact, many people with type 1 diabetes are afraid to start an exercise program because they fear the low blood sugar that comes from exercise dramatically enhancing their insulin sensitivity. Often this starts a cycle of getting hypoglycemic, treating the low blood sugar, and then becoming hyperglycemic; thus, the cycle of ups and downs begins. I'll be the first to say that exercising with type 1 diabetes is not easy. It's just not. There is definitely a learning curve in the beginning. Exercise with type 1 diabetes is not easy, but it is worth it!

If you are just starting an exercise program, make sure you discuss it with your diabetes health care team first. They may make adjustments in your insulin dosing or meal strategy. In addition, you may need to have testing done to make sure your body is ready to exercise. Once your doctor has given you the green light, you are all set to begin your routine. It should be approached like you are doing a science experiment. After all, you are introducing a new variable (exercise) and you want to know its effects. To do this, it may be helpful to exercise at the same time each day and for the same amount of time. What you want to do is figure out how your diabetes responds to exercise, so the more things you can keep constant, the easier it will be to figure out. You will want to keep a log of your data including time of day, blood sugar before, during, and after exercise, type of exercise, intensity of exercise, and amount of time spent exercising. After a few days, you should be able to work out a plan with your doctor.

As far as I know, there is no one "best" way to handle type 1 diabetes and exercise. If you start asking around, you will find all kinds of strategies for exercise. I'll share with you some of mine, but please discuss everything with your own doctor before trying it. I find it best to start planning exercise about 2 hours in advance if I can. I try to never exercise at a time when my last bolus of insulin is peaking. Depending on the type of short-acting insulin you are using, the peak will be between 2 to 4 hours. Since exercise has an insulin-like effect on glucose, exercising during the peak effect of insulin leads to a greater chance of a low blood sugar. When people without diabetes exercise, the level of insulin in their bloodstream is very low. I try to have a lower level of insulin on board to mimic nondiabetes physiology. To do this, I will often decrease my basal rate 30–45 minutes prior to exercise, during exercise, and up to a few hours after exercise depending on the intensity of the exercise and how long I did it. I find timing of exercise to be very useful. When exercising in the morning, usually there has been no bolus for several hours and this makes things a little easier. When exercising soon after a meal or snack, I will decrease the bolus I give for the meal or skip the bolus entirely for a snack that has 15–20 carbohydrates. Many people have suggested eating 15 grams of carbohydrates prior to exercise and 15–30 grams every 30 minutes during exercise with partial or no bolus depending on what my blood sugar is doing.

It is imperative to do frequent testing when you are starting an exercise routine or a new activity. Test before, during, and after exercise at the very least. I usually exercise with my continuous glucose monitor on, so it is easy for me to see trends. If you are exercising without one, test frequently so you know if you are 130 going up, 130 going down, or 130 holding steady. Once you get to know your body and how it handles certain exercises, you may not need to test as often as you do in the beginning.

Something that many people don't often think of is that intense exercise can actually increase blood sugar levels. While moderate exercise increases insulin sensitivity and increases glucose transport into cells from the bloodstream, strenuous exercise has the ability to increase blood glucose levels in the bloodstream. This is because strenuous exercise is a source of stress on the body. The sympathetic nervous system will be stimulated, and the fight or flight response is initiated. Our body doesn't know if we are in a spin class or being chased by a bear! The adrenal glands get busy releasing adrenaline into our systems and this stimulates glucose release. If the glucose released is more than the amount of glucose being used by our muscles, then the blood glucose levels will go up. How do we know when exercise will make our blood sugars go up instead of down? Strenuous exercise has been defined as exercise that is over 80% of our maximum exercise capacity, or our VO2max. This level usually corresponds with a heart rate that is over 90% of our maximum heart rate. If you can't talk at all to the person next to you, you are likely in this zone. I have read about people using intermittent bursts of vigorous activity, like sprinting for 60 seconds during an otherwise moderate run, to actually bump up their blood glucose to avoid getting low. I've never tried it myself, but it is an interesting concept.

To be safe, there are certain things we should all do when exercising with diabetes. The most important thing for anyone who runs a risk of becoming hypoglycemic is to have fast-acting carbohydrates immediately available. This could be glucose tablets, juice, Shot Bloks, Sport Beans, anything as long as it is rapidly absorbed into our system. Cheese and crackers won't cut it if you are dropping fast during a workout. If you are working out at a studio, gym, or at home, this is easy to do. Just have it in your gym bag. If you are out for a run or a hike, make sure that you have a way to carry the necessary supplies. I run with a Nathan runner's backpack. In it I carry my glucometer, my continuous glucose meter, rapid-acting glucose, a snack, my cell phone in case I need to call anyone, my ID, and money. People tease me and say I look like I'm going for a big adventure, but the way I see it, I'd rather be too prepared than be caught in a scary situation. This is the best backpack I've found because it securely straps down onto my body so things don't bounce around. I suggest trying a few different ways to carry your things with you so that you find the one that is the most comfortable.

Another thing that everyone with diabetes should have on them is a medical alert bracelet, card, or shoe tag, so that a stranger would easily be able to identify that you have diabetes. I also suggest that you work out with a partner who knows you have diabetes and knows how to treat a low blood sugar. This is particularly true if you are doing something remote like hiking or trail running. If you are in a spin class or dance class, take a moment before class starts to let the instructor know. You may be tempted to hide your diabetes, but letting people know is important, especially if the exercise is new to you.

With type 1 diabetes, there are definitely times when you should be cautious about exercise. The general guidelines are to check your blood glucose level and if it is over 250 and you are positive for ketones, do not exercise. To do so could potentially make things worse. If you have ketones, there is not enough insulin on board, and exercise may actually increase your blood sugar. If you are over 300, you should not exercise regardless if you have ketones or not. If you are less than 100, you should eat some carbohydrates and retest in 10 to 15 minutes.

Exercise with type 1 diabetes is a compromise. Unlike with type 2 diabetes, exercise may not actually improve your A1C. With the lows and highs that come with trying to balance insulin requirements, temporary basal rates, carbohydrate needs, etc., it can be a bumpy ride. However, even if your A1C doesn't budge at all, you are still reducing your risk of complications. Improved blood flow, improved cardiovascular fitness, improved blood pressure, increased metabolism, improved bone density, improved mood, improved sleep, and enhanced sense of well-being all still apply! And after the initial learning curve, things do get better. It's not easy, but it's worth it!

ⓙ SOUL-SEARCHING

Do you ever think that the "cost" (low blood sugars, planning required, etc.) of exercise isn't worth it?

_____

_____

_____

What benefits of exercise do you hope to add to your life? List three:

1. _____

2. _____

3. _____

HOW TO EXERCISE SAFELY WITH TYPE 1 AND TYPE 2 DIABETES

As women with diabetes, there are some particular areas that we need to pay attention to so that we make sure we exercise in the safest way possible. As I mentioned in the section for type 1 diabetes and exercise, when you start to exercise, you should exercise with someone who can recognize and treat a low blood sugar. You should always wear a medical alert tag to let people know you have diabetes, just in case. Always check your blood sugar before, during, and after exercise to make sure you know where your blood sugar is currently and where it's heading.

If you are new to exercise and considering starting an exercise routine, congratulations. Make sure you discuss it with your doctor. He or she may suggest some testing before you begin, to make sure you can do so safely. If there are any concerns about your heart health, you may need an EKG, a stress test, and/or an echo-cardiogram to make sure your heart is up to the task. If you have had diabetes for a long time, you are at increased risk for a "silent" heart attack, and you may not have the warning signs that often accompany heart disease. Your physician will want to rule this out. In addition, if you have peripheral neuropathy, you will need to pay special attention to your feet. Your doctor can help recommend shoes that will protect your feet during exercise. You will need good socks also to help prevent blisters from forming, as these can be entry points for bacteria to cause infection. You will need to check your feet every day to make sure you don't have any cuts, sores, or blisters that are forming. If you do, notify your physician. You will also need to be aware if you have peripheral vascular disease. If you have blood vessel disease to your legs, you may experience severe cramping with exercise. Again, discuss this with your doctor. If you have uncontrolled high blood pressure, your physician may want to get this under control before you do exercise. While exercise can help control blood pressure, in the

BE SAFE WHEN STARTING A NEW EXERCISE PROGRAM

- Tell your doctor
- Some people, especially those who have not been active for a while, may need a cardiac stress test
- Have eyes checked; if proliferative retinopathy is present, you may need to modify your exercise routine
- Be aware of peripheral neuropathy; wear the appropriate shoes and socks, and check your feet daily
- Make sure your blood pressure is not too high to safely exercise
- Check your blood glucose before, during, and after exercise
- Work out with someone who can recognize and treat low blood sugar
- Make sure you have rapid-acting carbohydrates immediately available

short term some exercises can actually raise it. If you are doing a strenuous workout, you need to be sure that your blood pressure is not going to be raised to a dangerous level. For the same reason, if you have diabetic proliferative retinopathy, your physician may suggest that you stay away from exercises that can increase the pressure in these blood vessels, like heavy lifting. You should have your eyes checked before starting a new exercise program so you can make changes in your exercise program to protect your eyes.

AVOIDING DEHYDRATION

Every person who exercises has to be aware of dehydration and how to prevent it, but if you are living with diabetes you really need to be aware. Water is vital in helping glucose or sugar move from where it is stuck in the bloodstream to where we need it to give us energy in our muscles. When we exercise, muscles use up their glucose stores, glycogen, and then depend on getting glucose from the bloodstream to supply them with energy. If the water content in your body is too low, the glucose stays in the bloodstream, and high blood sugar results. To make matters worse, high blood sugars cause your kidneys to make more urine and you end up losing even more water! This worsens dehydration, and thus the feedback loop has begun. If you follow a low-carb diet, you are more likely to experience dehydration due to the fluid loss that low-carb diets initiate.

Clues that you are dehydrated include feeling thirsty, feeling weak or tired, having nausea, cramping in the muscles, making less urine, and making very dark, concentrated urine.

There is some debate about how to best replenish your body with fluids. When considering using water versus using sports drinks that also replace electrolytes, there are a few things to keep in mind. Most experts agree that if you are exercising 1 hour or less, you are most likely fine replenishing with plain, old water. It's unlikely that you've lost really significant amounts of sodium or potassium in that time frame unless the conditions are extreme. On the other hand, if you will be exercising for more than 1 hour, you may want to use a sports drink that has electrolytes in it.

Beware of hidden problems, though. Many of these sports drinks are high in sugar and are packed with calories. Make sure you take these carbohydrates into account when you are planning out your exercise. The drinks can be a handy source of carbohydrates you need for exercise, just make sure you know exactly what you are getting. I find it useful to have a sports drink and water. If I am thirsty but my blood sugar is normal to high, I will drink water. If I notice that I'm dropping or on the lower end of the spectrum, I will use the sports drink to bump things up. Many people choose to dilute the sports drink with water to cut the calories and sugar in half. Talk with your diabetes team to plan a strategy that works for you.

OVERCOME COMMON BARRIERS TO EXERCISE AND HAVE FUN IN THE PROCESS

Okay, so by now you probably know you should be exercising. You know all the health benefits, you know that you will feel better, but there still might be something holding you back. One of the most common barriers to overcome is simply finding the time. No matter what phase of life you are in, most women carry insane schedules. Between bills, doctor's appointments, work, family, pets, etc., it might feel like there is no time left for you to do anything for yourself. If you feel like you just can't make time for exercise, I suggest scheduling exercise appointments. Put exercise in your daily calendar just like you would for a dentist appointment or your child's soccer practice. Exercise is not an optional thing to do only if you have time. You will never have time. You have to make time for what is important, and exercise is important. Schedule it early in the day so that you are less likely to have unplanned circumstances pop up and ruin your schedule. It also helps if you schedule it with a friend. There have been many times when the only thing that made me show up for my exercise class was the fact that someone was there waiting for me.

If you are just too busy, see if you can work your exercise into other daily routines. Walk to the dry cleaner or to the grocery store. Every little bit of exercise counts. Another strategy is to have fallback exercises for those really busy days. If you plan on going to the gym or on a run every day, but just run out of time, have an alternative. Keep a jump rope at home: This is a great cardiovascular exercise and requires little space. If you live in a building, climb up and down the stairs. Have a couple of workout DVDs that you have in your living room that you can do if you need to exercise at odd hours. Having a backup plan will help you meet your 150 minutes per week no matter what your schedule looks like.

Another common barrier to exercise is the feeling that it's just too hard or unpleasant. This happens when too much is attempted too quickly. Remember, start nice and slow. This will not only be good for your body, but you are much more likely to stick to your exercise plan if you don't feel like you are about to pass out the entire time. As for the feeling miserable part, no one ever said exercise had to be unpleasant. If you hate running, don't run! If I had to run every day, I'd probably exercise once every 2 weeks. It's important to find something that you actually enjoy doing so that you look forward to it. For me, I love spin class. I like the music, I like the atmosphere, and I like seeing friends there. I sometimes go just for the social aspect or to feel like I've gone out dancing. Hula hooping is a great way to work your core and is making a comeback. Trapeze class can offer a wonderful workout for your arms; I know from experience. Try taking a salsa dance class with your best friend. Start a garden in your backyard and commit to working in it for 30 minutes each day. Make exercise fun! You'll enjoy it more and be more likely to stick to it.

Being overly focused on specific outcomes can give us motivation, but can also backfire. If you are only exercising to decrease your A1C or to lose weight, you are likely to fall off track if these numbers don't budge. Don't focus on outcomes; focus on the moment. Tune in to how you feel after exercise. If you are in a bad mood, instead of reaching for the cookies, reach for your tennis shoes. Even 5 minutes of walking will improve your mood. If you focus on how you feel after exercise, you will be more likely to stick to it. Exercise to exercise. Remember all of the benefits that it offers to you, no matter what the scale or the lab results say! You are so much more than a number, a glucose value, or a size.

None of those things can measure the years you are adding on to your life, the sense of well-being you are creating, or the social bonds you are strengthening when you exercise.

When all else fails, don't be afraid to use a cute outfit to get you excited. I know it sounds crazy, but having those too-cute running shoes, those new hot pink sweatpants, or a fun new headband can be the motivation you need to get out the door. When I won *The Amazing Race,* one of my splurges was on Lululemon workout tops. They are so cute, have fun little pockets to hide glucose and meters in, and just made me feel like a yoga diva/athlete. I wanted to work out so I had an excuse to wear my fun new threads! Use whatever it takes, but don't be afraid to tap into that part of you that loves to shop/wear glitter/tutus, etc. It's a powerful force; use it to your advantage!

 SOUL-SEARCHING

What are some things you can do to get more excited about exercise?

_____

_____

_____

Do you have any friends or groups that would start an exercise routine with you?

_____

_____

 NOTES ON MY JOURNEY

_____

_____

_____

Navigating Your Career

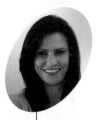

BRANDY SAYS...

One summer job I took during college made a lasting impression on me, and it wasn't positive. The job only lasted for 2 months, but I learned a lot about the world. I was 20 at the time and I had a long life ahead of me, so I thought. The owner of the business was in his 60s or 70s and was also very "old school" in his thinking. He came in while I was working one day and he overheard a conversation I was having with another employee about my diabetes. The owner looked at me, shocked, and asked, "How old are you?" I told him. "Well, your life is already a third over because you'll be dead by 60. So you'd better get to livin'," he said.

Shocked at his audacity and lack of empathy, I stood there speechless. They say that the negative comments stick with you more so than positive ones, and in this case, I agree. I had never once thought about how much time I had "left" to live. His perspective is a great example of looking at the glass as half empty. Up until then, I had always been focused on achieving and accomplishing and how I was going to get that done. I still wish he had never poisoned my positive thoughts with his negative one. I still find myself thinking about it every once in a while.

While what my former employer said is crude and ignorant, his comments alone did not break any laws because I was not discriminated against due to my diabetes. If his comments had been followed by a refusal to hire me as a full-time employee a few months later or a refusal to allow me to take breaks to check my blood sugar, then the possibility of discrimination could have been pursued.

Most often, workplace discrimination is the result of an employer's ignorance or belief in stereotypes. While the issue of employment rights often seems complicated and cumbersome, there are some basic guidelines that anyone with diabetes who is or wants to become gainfully employed should familiarize oneself with.

LAWS THAT PROTECT YOU

First, it pays to know what laws are in place to protect you. Since 1994, the Americans with Disabilities Act (ADA) has covered all private and state/local government-based employees with disabilities who are employed in companies with more than 15 employees. Specifically, the ADA "prohibits discrimination in all employment practices including job application procedures, hiring, firing, advancement, compensation, training, and other terms, conditions, and privileges of employment. It applies to recruitment, advertising, tenure, layoff, fringe benefits, and all other employment-related activities." The **Rehabilitation Act of 1973** generally covers employees who work for the executive branch of the federal government, or any employee who receives federal money. The **Congressional Accountability Act** covers employees of Congress and most legislative branch agencies. In addition, all states have their own anti-discrimination laws in effect. Some are more comprehensive than others. Check with your state government for more detailed information.

Secondly, it's important to understand what qualifies you for protection under these laws. In order to be protected by federal anti-discrimination laws, a worker must show that she is a "qualified individual with a disability." There are actually two parts to this qualification. First, a qualified individual is one who satisfies the skill, experience, education, and other job-related requirements of the position held or desired and who—if given reasonable accommodation—can fulfill the essential functions of the position. The next step is to establish that the worker has a disability, a record of a disability, or is regarded as having a disability. A disability is defined as a mental or physical impairment that substantially limits one or more major life activities, such as eating, walking, seeing, or caring for oneself. It also could apply to a person whose body has trouble, unassisted, with a major physical function (such as a compromised endocrine system). A person with diabetes would be assessed under the parameters of these laws without considering mitigating measures, such as insulin.

> "I firmly believe in the rule of law as the foundation for all of our basic rights."
>
> *Sonia Sotomayor, Supreme Court Justice, who lives with diabetes*

YOUR RIGHTS IN THE WORKPLACE

Over the years, I have received countless questions from women with diabetes regarding their rights in the workplace. From medical leave, to being terminated, to eating snacks at work, I have heard it all. Below are some basic rights that all women with diabetes should be aware of:

Questions About Your Diabetes

During the interview process, potential employers cannot ask about your medical conditions or the prescription medications you use. If an applicant voluntarily tells an employer that she has diabetes during the interview process, the employer may only ask two questions: Do you need a reasonable accommodation? And if so, what type of accommodation do you need? The fact that an applicant has diabetes may not be used to withdraw a job offer if the applicant is able to perform the fundamental duties of the job, with or without reasonable accommodation, and without posing a direct threat to her safety.

Physical Exams

Potential employers cannot require you to submit to a physical exam during the interview process. However, once an employment offer has been extended, employers can require to you submit to a physical exam, as long as it is a standard requirement for all employees.

In addition, your employer can require you to undergo a physical exam when you make a request for reasonable accommodations, when you return from an extended medical leave, or when you experience a problem on the job (such as severe or repetitive hypoglycemia).

Safety Issues

Employers sometimes use the "direct threat" defense when faced with discrimination charges. When this is used, the employer believes that the employee would pose a "direct threat" or significant risk of substantial harm to herself or others that cannot be reduced or eliminated through reasonable accommodations. To use this defense, the employer must have completed an assessment on the individual based on objective, factual evidence, including the best recent medical evidence and advances to control and treat diabetes.

Medical Leave

The Family Medical Leave Act (FMLA) is a law that protects workers who must miss work due to their own serious health condition or to care for a family member, such as a child, spouse, or parent. Diabetes qualifies as a serious condition if it requires that you go to the doctor at least twice a year or if it requires hospitalization. To qualify, you must have worked for the same employer for 12 consecutive months and for 1,250 hours during those 12 months of employment. Your employer must also have at leave 50 employees within 75 miles of each other.

If you fit the above qualifications, your employer is required to allow you to take up to 12 weeks of unpaid leave. This leave can be taken all at once, for example, 12 weeks back-to-back, or it can be broken up into smaller chunks (for doctor appointments, etc.).

For FMLA approval, you and your physician will have to complete the paperwork provided by your employer within 15 days of receiving it. Once you have used the 12 weeks of FMLA leave, your employer is not required to allow you to take any more unpaid leave.

Hypoglycemia

You cannot be fired for having an episode of hypoglycemia without your employer first conducting an individual assessment to determine safety risk, and without considering whether there are any reasonable accommodations that could eliminate the safety risk. This assessment may include a medical evaluation. However, if you violate a workplace conduct rule due to inappropriate behavior caused by a low blood sugar, you employer has the right to discipline you.

Termination

Being fired, or let go, from a job is usually a traumatic experience. It's even worse if you think it happened because of discriminatory actions from your employer due to your diabetes. If you think your termination is due to your diabetes, allow yourself to cool off for a few days before pursuing legal action. When you are ready to talk about it, contact the American Diabetes Association to speak with an attorney who is highly knowledgeable about how to pursue such cases successfully.

IS THIS JOB A GOOD FIT FOR YOU AND YOUR DIABETES?

- Before going on a job interview, do your research to find out what kind, if any, of health insurance is offered. If possible, talk to a current employee to find out about deductibles and coverage for prescription medications (diabetes pills, insulin, etc.) and medical devices (insulin pumps, continuous glucose monitors, etc.). Research the company online or talk to current employees if possible. Insurance can, and often is, the selling factor of a job for single women with diabetes. It is very difficult to survive financially without health insurance.

- After going on a job interview, assess every aspect (work schedule, work flow, sick leave policy) to not only assess if you can and would enjoy the work, but to determine if it would be a good fit for you and your diabetes. For example, if you are considering a job as a receptionist at a busy doctor's office and they have told you up front that lunchtime is inconsistent from day-to-day and some days you may not get a lunch, it may not be a good fit for you and your diabetes.

- Many health insurance plans now offer chronic illness programs that provide educational materials, preventive reminders, and access to a personal health manager. Check to see if the company where you are interviewing offers this benefit.

REASONABLE ACCOMMODATIONS

Reasonable accommodations are changes that enable qualified applicants or employees with disabilities to participate in the application process or to perform essential job junctions. They also include adjustments to ensure that qualified individuals with disabilities have rights and privileges in employment that are equal to those of employees without disabilities. Such accommodations for people with diabetes are mandated by federal anti-discrimination laws, unless doing so would create an undue hardship (i.e., a significant difficulty or expense). Your employer may have to change an otherwise valid workplace policy for you. You cannot be denied a reasonable accommodation just because it goes against standard policies or because non-disabled employees are not entitled to it. Accommodations vary depending on the needs of each individual. Not all people with diabetes will need an accommodation or will require the same accommodation.

Some of the common reasonable accommodations for individuals with diabetes include:

- a private area to test blood glucose or administer insulin
- the ability to keep diabetes supplies and food nearby
- the ability to test blood glucose and inject insulin anywhere at work
- a place to rest until blood sugar levels become normal
- breaks to check blood glucose levels, eat snacks, take medication, or go to the restroom
- a modified work schedule or shift change
- the ability to leave work for treatment, recuperation, or training for managing diabetes (this may also fall under the Family and Medical Leave Act)
- modifications to no-fault attendance policies
- appropriate containers for needles/syringe disposal
- frequent breaks for food as needed
- appropriate food for office-sponsored events and reward programs
- modifications to policies involving food storage and consumption
- removal of temperature extremes to help deal with poor circulation
- opportunities to educate coworkers on emergency situation procedures and identification of symptoms of hypoglycemia or hyperglycemia

- modification of job tasks that require fine finger dexterity, to accommodate neuropathy
- anti-fatigue mats or padded carpeting for neuropathy issues
- flexibility to sit or stand to accommodate neuropathy

There are certainly other reasonable accommodations that can be requested. It is important for you and your employer to discuss your individual needs. To request a reasonable accommodation, you simply need to talk with your employer about how to meet your needs. Although a written request is not required, I am a firm believer in documentation of such matters, especially when there are so many documented cases of discrimination. Better safe than sorry. A written request also provides clarification of your request and how it will help you perform your job. Be prepared to provide documentation of your disability and the need for your accommodation from your health care provider. There is no need to provide additional information beyond this. In fact, there are strict limitations on what information your employer is permitted to request. Your health care provider should not communicate with your employer without your permission and he or she should primarily communicate in writing rather than by phone so that there is a written record of the conversation. You should also keep a detailed record of all communication with your employer on this matter, including conversations, emails, and voicemails. Be open to suggestions from and negotiations with your employers, but be clear about what will and will not work. If you or your employer are unsure about a suggested accommodation option, propose a trial period to assess its viability.

It is completely up to you whether or not you disclose your diabetes diagnosis to your employer or coworkers. There is no requirement that you tell prospective or current employers that you have diabetes, for most types of jobs. In jobs that require certain skills or abilities, such as commercial driving, in which a serious diabetes complication might prevent you from doing the job (or could cause you harm), you must disclose that you have diabetes.

But no matter what you decide, you must know that in order for you to qualify as having a disability under the Americans with Disabilities Act, you have to acknowledge that you have diabetes. Also, while there are unique cases where people have decided it is not in their best interest to disclose their diabetes, for the most part it is best to be open about your diabetes. That way, those around you can help if an emergency situation arises. You may still choose to only disclose the information you feel is necessary for them to assist you. Again, you are not required to answer any questions.

SOUL-SEARCHING

Have you ever experienced or witnessed disability discrimination at work? What happened?

_____

_____

_____

_____

_____

Based on what you learned in this chapter, was it handled properly? If not, how should it have been handled?

_____

_____

_____

_____

_____

_____

TIPS FOR BETTER DIABETES MANAGEMENT AT WORK

- Keep snacks in many places: in your desk, the kitchen, your purse, your computer bag, etc. Careful planning will help prevent embarrassing and untimely low blood sugar situations.

- Balancing work, healthy eating, exercise, and blood sugar testing can be difficult at times. In busy times, it's easier to grab an unhealthy snack or meal because it's close by. Avoid this unhealthy habit by planning your lunches and snacks at the beginning of the week. If you have healthy foods at your desk, there's no reason to go to the vending machine.

- Try to identify at least one person at your workplace (preferably someone who is close to you during most of the workday) with whom you can comfortably disclose your diabetes. Having at least one person who knows what symptoms to look for with low and high blood sugars and how to treat them is critical to your health.

- Keep extra diabetes supplies at work: an extra meter, test strips, pump supplies, insulin, medications. This will prevent unnecessary trips back home to retrieve forgotten supplies.

- Start the workday off right; don't skip breakfast.

- To avoid widely fluctuating or high blood sugars in the morning (which will often result in sluggishness), don't eat a high-carbo-hydrate meal before work.

LIFE APPLICATION

Based on what you've read in this chapter, what steps can you take today to better protect yourself in the workplace?

_____

_____

_____

RESTRICTED JOBS

Thanks to the Americans with Disabilities Act and organizations like the American Diabetes Association, which have fought to end employment discrimination, there aren't many jobs that are off-limits to women with diabetes. Over the past decade, fitness guidelines have been adapted for fire fighters, police officers, and other law enforcement personnel so that each individual applicant can be assessed for competency; no longer are people with diabetes automatically banned from these jobs. In addition, people who used insulin once could not be commercial drivers; now they may hold these positions if they obtain a Department of Transportation medical certification. The only careers that are not open to people with diabetes (those who require insulin) are first-class commercial pilots and certain military jobs. We've come a long way, baby!

MY DIABETES JOURNAL

What stresses me out the most about managing my diabetes in the workplace is:

_____

_____

_____

NOTES ON MY JOURNEY

_____

_____

_____

Although this book is coming to an end, that doesn't mean that our time together has to be over. Peer support and education have been shown to have a very positive impact on the health and well-being of women with diabetes. If you learned something new from this book, I encourage you to share it with others. Not only is it important for us to do our part to educate the public about diabetes and its unique impact on women, but it's up to us to come together as a strong sisterhood to support, encourage, and educate each other. Without this kind of unity, we are just millions of women trying to figure out this disease all alone. Strength is found in numbers and the sisterhood needs you!

RESOURCES

DIABETES AND EMPLOYMENT RESOURCES

Thomas, V., JD, and Lorber, D., MD, FACP, CDE: Diabetes Goes to Work. *Practical Diabetology,* Vol. 28, no. 4, 2009 (November/December).

American Diabetes Association
www.diabetes.org

Americans with Disabilities Act Amendments Act
http://www.eeoc.gov/laws/statutes/adaaa_info.cfm

EEOC and Diabetes Discrimination
http://www.eeoc.gov/laws/types/diabetes.cfm

RESOURCES FOR WOMEN WITH DIABETES

American Diabetes Association's Women's Initiative
The mission of the Women's Initiative is to provide education and support for women who are at risk for diabetes, who live with diabetes, and/or who care for family members with diabetes.
www.diabetes.org/women

DiabetesSisters
DiabetesSisters is a 501(c)3 national nonprofit organization whose mission is to improve the health and quality of life of women with

diabetes and those at risk of developing diabetes, as well as to advocate on their behalf. Signature programming includes the DiabetesSisters' Conference Series, the PODS Meetups program, and the Life Class Webinar Series. The organization's website also offers a variety of online resources such as Expert Advice articles, sisterTALK blogs, and the Women's Forum.

www.diabetessisters.org • **info@diabetessisters.org**
919-361-2012

Juvenile Diabetes Research Foundation Pregnancy Toolkit

Pregnancy or planning a pregnancy with type 1 diabetes requires special consideration to help ensure a healthy outcome for mother and child. This guide provides information for parents-to-be or future parents-to-be with type 1 diabetes—explaining disease management goals for pregnancy and reviewing how to obtain the best possible support from health care providers at every stage.

http://jdrf.org/life-with-t1d/pregnancy/

Society for Women's Health Research (SWHR)

SWHR is the thought leader in research on biological differences in disease and is dedicated to transforming women's health through science, advocacy, and education. Founded in 1990 by a group of physicians, medical researchers, and health advocates, SWHR aims to bring attention to the variety of diseases and conditions that uniquely affect women. Thanks to efforts of SWHR, women are now routinely included in most major medical research studies, and scientists are considering gender as a variable in their research.

http://womenshealthresearch.org

Centers for Disease Control and Prevention

The Centers for Disease Control and Prevention is currently focused on implementing interventions to improve access and quality of care for women with a history of gestational diabetes through collaborations with national and state partners.

http://www.cdc.gov/diabetes/projects/women.htm

U.S. Food and Drug Administration (FDA)

http://www.fda.gov/ForConsumers/ByAudience/ForWomen/
WomensHealthTopics/ucm117969.htm

International Diabetes Federation's Women's Program
The mission of the International Diabetes Federation is to promote diabetes care, prevention, and a cure worldwide.

http://www.idf.org/women-and-diabetes

FDA's Office of Women's Health

www.Womenshealth.gov

DIABETES AND EATING DISORDERS RESOURCES

We Are Diabetes
We Are Diabetes is an organization primarily devoted to promoting support and awareness for people with type 1 diabetes who suffer from eating disorders. We are dedicated to providing guidance, hope and resources to those who may be struggling, as well as to their families and loved ones.

We Are Diabetes also advocates for living well and living strong with type 1 diabetes. The daily challenges of living with this disease, as well as the emotional and financial toll it takes, can oftentimes result in a sense of defeat or isolation. We help those who feel alone in their chronic illness find hope and courage to live healthy, happy lives!

http://www.wearediabetes.org

Diabulimia Helpline
The Diabulimia Hotline is the country's only nonprofit organization dedicated to education, support, and advocacy for diabetic individuals with eating disorders and their loved ones. A 24-hour hotline is available (425-985-3635), an insurance specialist is available to walk clients or their loved ones through the complicated world of insurance coverage, and there is a referral service

to help people find the right treatment center, doctor, and/or therapist that will be a good fit on the road to recovery.

http://www.diabulimiahelpline.org/

EATING DISORDER TREATMENT CENTERS

Center for Hope of the Sierras
Located in Reno, Nevada, the Center for Hope's diabulimia program is focused on the biology of eating disorders and diabetes as well as the psychological, social, and cultural implications that are interwoven into the biological process. With treatment anchored in the biopsychosocial model, women in the diabulimia program receive: comprehensive medical management, including nutritional education and rehabilitation; blood sugar monitoring/testing; insulin re-introduction; a monitored exercise program; individual, group, and family therapy, which addresses the food, weight, body image, and interpersonal issues underlying an eating disorder as well as the emotional factors that are interfering with responsible self-care. This center offers 24-hour nursing and social support.

http://www.centerforhopeofthesierras.com
866-690-7242

Park Nicollet Melrose Institute
Located in St. Louis Park, Minneapolis, the Melrose Institute collaborates with the International Diabetes Center at Park Nicollet to treat people struggling with the dual diagnosis of an eating disorder and type 1 diabetes. Care teams include a pediatric and adult endocrinologist, psychiatrist, psychologist, diabetes nurse educator, and diabetes nutrition educator. A care manager helps coordinate treatment, keeps communication consistent, and answers questions for patients and families.

http://www.parknicollet.com/eatingdisorders/
800-862-7412

Eating Recovery Center

Located in Denver, Colorado, Eating Recovery Center is a licensed hospital facility with a 24-hour nursing staff and daily visits from a medical doctor, which creates an environment that can accommodate most health complications that arise. The program also offers a family therapy program that can incorporate the whole family into the healing process. There are two separate on-site facilities to accommodate adolescent and adult patients.

http://www.eatingrecoverycenter.com
Info@EatingRecoveryCenter.com
877-825-8584

Cumberland Hospital for Children and Adolescents

Located in New Kent, Virginia, Cumberland Hospital patients who are living with both diabetes and an eating disorder participate in a specially designed diabetes program that is now recognized by the American Diabetes Association. Adolescents with diabetes learn and practice healthy eating and exercise habits, as well as cooking skills and medication management. They participate in Cumberland's EAT (Eating Attitudes Training) group, learning to make healthy choices in the cafeteria and at restaurants. The program also addresses issues such as body image, nutrition and positive attitudes and helps adolescents change their distorted thinking patterns. During family therapy, families learn healthy ways to help their child and live with their child's disease.

http://cumberlandhospital.com/chronic-illness/diabetes-and-
    eating-disorders/
Kent.Hugill@uhsinc.com
800-368-3472

GENERAL DIABETES RESOURCES

American Diabetes Association

The Association's mission is to prevent and cure diabetes and to improve the lives of all people affected by diabetes. The moving force behind the work of the Association is a network of more than 1 million volunteers, a membership of more than 441,000 people with diabetes and their families and caregivers, a professional society of nearly 16,500 health care professionals, and more than 800 staff members.

www.diabetes.org

Behavioral Diabetes Institute (BDI)

BDI, a 501(c)(3) nonprofit organization located in San Diego, California, focuses on addressing the social, emotional, and psychological barriers to living a long and healthy life with diabetes. To better understand and overcome these obstacles, BDI is actively engaged in research examining the psychological aspects of diabetes and evaluating innovative behavioral interventions. In addition, BDI directly offers an array of unique, behaviorally oriented products and services for the following: people with type 1 diabetes, people with type 2 diabetes, parents of children and teens with diabetes, spouses and partners of people with diabetes, and interested health care professionals.

www.behavioraldiabetes.org

FDA Patient Network

Created in 2012, the FDA Patient Network is part of the Office of Health and Constituent Affairs (OHCA), formerly the Office of Special Health Issues. They work to help patients, patient advocates, and their health care professionals connect with FDA science and policy staff.

http://patientnetwork.fda.gov/

GENERAL HEALTH RESOURCES FOR WOMEN

HealthyWomen/National Women's Health Resource Center

HealthyWomen (HW) is the nation's leading independent health information source for women. Their core mission is to educate, inform, and empower women to make smart health choices for themselves and their families. For more than 20 years, millions of women have gone to HW for answers to their most pressing and personal health care questions. Through a wide array of online and print publications, HW provides health information that is original, objective, reviewed by medical experts, and reflective of the advances in evidence-based health research.

www.healthywomen.org

National Women's Health Network
The National Women's Health Network seeks to improve the health of all women by developing and promoting a critical analysis of health issues and aspires to a health care system that is guided by social justice to reflect the needs of diverse women.

www.nwhn.org

The U.S. Department of Health and Human Services: Office on Women's Health
The Office on Women's Health is a project of the U.S. Department of Health and Human Services' Office of Women's Health (OWH). The OWH provides national leadership and coordination to improve the health of women and girls through policy, education, and model programs.

www.womenshealth.gov

ONLINE DIABETES SUPPORT NETWORKS

www.diabetessisters.org
www.tudiabetes.org
www.diabeteshandsfoundation.org
www.diabetesdaily.com

WOMEN'S REPRODUCTIVE/SEXUAL HEALTH RESOURCES

American College of Obstetricians and Gynecologists (ACOG)

The American College of Obstetricians and Gynecologists is the nation's leading group of professionals providing health care for women.

www.acog.org

National Vulvodynia Association

The National Vulvodynia Association (NVA) is a nonprofit organization dedicated to improving the lives of individuals affected by vulvodynia, a spectrum of chronic vulvar pain disorders.

www.nva.org

American Menopause Foundation

This foundation is a nonprofit health organization providing support and assistance on all issues concerning menopause.

www.americanmenopause.org

North American Menopause Society

The North American Menopause Society is the leading nonprofit scientific organization devoted to promoting women's health and quality of life through an understanding of menopause.

www.menopause.org

Red Hot Mamas

Red Hot Mamas® is the leading provider of menopause education and support programs in the United States and Canada and has been educating and engaging women, and health care providers, since 1991. The organization has focused solely on providing information and support to women to help optimize their health at menopause and beyond.

www.redhotmamas.org

American Association of Sexuality Educators, Counselors, and Therapists

The American Association of Sexuality Educators, Counselors, and Therapists is a nonprofit organization that promotes understanding of human sexuality and healthy sexual behavior.

www.aasect.org

Kinsey Institute for Research in Sex, Gender, and Reproduction

The mission of the Kinsey Institute is to promote interdisciplinary research and scholarship in the fields of human sexuality, gender, and reproduction.

www.kinseyinstitute.org

National Sexuality Resource Center

This center gathers and disseminates the latest information and research on sexual health, education, and rights.

www.nsrc.sfsu.edu

UCLA Women's Health Center

The Iris Cantor UCLA Women's Health Education & Resource Center mission is to provide comprehensive, exemplary health education programs to women and their loved ones that inform, support, and empower women to achieve their optimal level of health.

Womenshealth.ucla.edu

His and Her Health

HisandHerHealth.com is a website providing information about both men and women, and includes a sexual health forum and many articles on sexual health. It also includes the latest highlights in sexual health news.

www.hisandherhealth.com

Urology Care Foundation

The Urology Care Foundation is committed to promoting urology research and education. We work with researchers, health care professionals, patients, and caregivers to improve patients' lives. The Urology Care Foundation is the official foundation of the American Urological Association (AUA)—an organization of roughly 20,000 urologists.

www.urologyhealth.org

Female Sexual Dysfunction Online

This website provides clinicians and researchers with factual, accurate, and balanced educational materials regarding female sexual dysfunction.

www.femalesexualdysfunctiononline.org

INDEX